Midwives
AND *Safer*
Motherhood

EDITOR

Susan F. Murray

MA (Hons) Sociology, RN, RM

Lecturer in Maternal Health,
Centre for International Child Health,
Institute of Child Health, London

FOREWORD

Dr Tomris Türmen

Executive Director, Family and Reproductive Health,
World Health Organization, Geneva

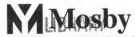

Mosby

London Baltimore Barcelona Bogotá Boston Buenos Aires Caracas Carlsbad, CA Chicago Madrid Mexico City Milan Naples, FL New York Philadelphia St. Louis Seoul Singapore Sydney Tair

Mosby titles of related interest:
Jones: *Ethics in Midwifery*, 1994
Richardson & Webber: *Ethical Issues in Child Health Care*, 1996
Dimond: *The Legal Aspects of Child Health Care*, 1996
Campbell & Glasper: *Whaley and Wong's Children's Nursing*, 1995

Project Manager:	Dave Burin
Cover Design/Designer:	Lara Last
Production:	Mike Heath
Layout Artist:	John Ormiston
Illustration:	Marion Tasker
Cover Illustration:	Deborah Gyan
Development Editor:	Hannah Tudge
Publisher:	Griselda Campbell

Published by Mosby, an imprint of Times Mirror International Publishers Limited

Printed in England by J W Arrowsmith Ltd

ISBN 0 7234 2122 6

For full details of all Times Mirror International Publishers Limited titles, please write to Times Mirror International Publishers Limited, Lynton House, 7–12 Tavistock Square, London WC1H 9LB, England.

A CIP catalogue record for this book is available from the British Library.

Contents

Contributors

Gloria A. Betts is a midwifery teacher with many years of experience. She is the former principal of the National School of Midwifery in Sierra Leone and immediate past Chairperson of the West African College of Nursing – MCH Faculty. She has been the International Confederation of Midwives Regional Representative for Africa since 1987 and was a founding and executive member of the Sierra Leone Midwives Association. She has been an advisor to the Sierra Leone Government, to UNICEF and to the World Health Organization. In 1993 and 1994 she was a member of the WHO Global Advisory Group on Nursing and Midwifery.

Grace E. Delano is a Fellow of the West African College of Nursing, and Executive Director/Vice President of the Association for Reproductive and Family Health in Nigeria. She has a long history of work in the field of reproductive health and family planning. She has served as a member of a World Health Organization (WHO) Advisory Committee to review guidelines for the treatment of unsafe abortion, and as a reproductive health consultant to numerous international organizations. She has written extensively, and in 1993 received the WHO Sasakawe Health Award.

Raymond G. DeVries is Associate Professor of Sociology, St. Olaf College in Northfield, Minnesota and is author of *Regulating Birth: Midwives, Medicine and the Law*. His interest in midwifery is part of a wider concern with the influence of law and professionalisation on health care. His recent research includes an examination of the history and current status of midwives in the Netherlands, and sociological analysis of the new profession of bioethicist.

Marie-Claude Foster is Lecturer in Management at the Centre for International Child Health (University of London). She has training in sociology, preventive health and education, and has extensive experience in social science research. She writes, teaches, and provides consultancy on organizational development, group processes, stress in organizations, and on the management of change.

Charlotte E. Hord is a Program and Policy Associate with IPAS (International Projects Assistance Services) in North Carolina, USA, a non-governmental agency dedicated to improving reproductive health care. She collaborates with Ministry of Health policy makers, individual health professionals, and representatives of non-governmental organizations to develop and implement strategies for improving the quality and management of abortion care. Recently, she headed an assessment of the potential for involving midwives and other non-physicians in IPAS' work, and served as a co-author for a WHO manual on post-abortion family planning.

Barbara E. Kwast is a midwife educator and epidemiologist. Until recently she was Maternal and Neonatal Health Advisor for the MotherCare Project, John Snow Inc., USA. She worked in Africa between 1965 and 1986, as a midwife tutor in Malawi and Nigeria and as Lecturer in Community Obstetrics in the Department of Obstetrics and Gynaecology of the University of Addis Ababa, Black Lion Hospital, Ethiopia. From 1986 to 1991 she worked with WHO, Geneva in maternal and perinatal mortality research, as a member of a UNFPA interregional team and in the WHO Safe Motherhood Initiative, She is presently involved with national programmes on implementation, evaluation and research in safe motherhood in Africa, Asia and Latin America.

Marta J. Levitt, is a medical anthropologist. She is the MCH/FP Advisor to Redd Barna (South Asia) and advisor to the National TBA Programme, Ministry of Health, Nepal. For the past 18 years she has been conducting research and implementing projects on women and health. She has worked in Hawaii, the Philippines, Taiwan, Nepal, and Bhutan. From 1986–1987 she was principal Investigator for 'A Systematic Study of Birth and Traditional Birth Attendants in Nepal'. She also helped develop the Safe Home Delivery Kit for Nepal.

Maureen Minden is the MCH Coordinator for the American Refugee Committee Burmese Border Program in Thailand. She is a midwife, with a background in education and social anthropology. In the 1970s and 1980s she was involved in efforts to include midwifery as a profession in the Canadian health care system, a goal just now being realized. In 1986 she moved to the UK where she practised in the National Health Service. From 1989 to 1992 she was responsible for Mother and Child Health and for TBA training in the Kavre District of Nepal with Voluntary

Service Overseas (VSO), and in 1993 she completed an MSc in Mother and Child Health at the Institute of Child Health, University of London. She is co-author of the English-language edition of Nepal's TBA training and supervision manual.

Susan F. Murray is Lecturer in Maternal Health at the Centre for International Child Health, Institute of Child Health (University of London). She has training in midwifery, sociology and education. Her past experience includes hospital midwifery, administration of a mobile clinic, and coordination of a clinical trial, and from 1987 to 1990 she worked in Nicaragua in TBA training, active birth education, and education for reproductive health. She teaches and writes on Safe Motherhood issues and has travelled extensively. Her current research concerns the social construction of birth by caesarean section in Chile.

Esnart Shakulipa Namakando trained as a registered nurse and midwife at the University Teaching Hospital, Lusaka, Zambia. She worked as staff nurse/midwife as well as clinical teacher before pursuing her post-basic nursing studies at the University of Zambia and the University of London. She has worked as midwifery teacher at the University Teaching Hospital School of Midwifery since 1985. She has also participated in national MCH programme evaluation. Since 1988, she has also been involved in reproductive health research in the Department of Obstetrics and Gynaecology, University of Zambia.

Susan Ama Opoku is the research coordinator for the Ashanti Region Health Services, Ghana. She worked as a public health nurse in the MCH/FP Division from 1989–1992. In 1993 she completed postgraduate studies in MCH at the Institute of Child Health in London. She is particularly interested in health systems research and has been a team member of the Prevention of Maternal Mortality Network in West Africa since 1989.

Abimbola Olufunmilola Payne is a Registered Health Service Administrator, and is currently Resident Advisor, MotherCare Nigeria, Lagos, Nigeria. She has served as Chief Nursing Officer/Advisor to the Federal Ministry of Health, and spent 25 years teaching midwifery and training nurse/midwife tutors. She also helped to initiate the National Programme on the training of Traditional Birth Attendants. She was Chair of the Faculty of Maternal and Child Health and Member of Council of the West African College of Nursing for 4 years. She is a member of the Society of Gynaecologists and Obstetricians of Nigeria's National Task Force on Safe Motherhood, and of the Women's Health Organisation of Nigeria.

Patricia Semeraro is a certified nurse-midwife currently working at the Rockville Center, New York. She has been a midwife consultant to the Population Council for the last 8 years, working on various breastfeeding and postpartum projects. She is a co-author of the Population Council publication, *Contraception during breastfeeding: A Clinician's Sourcebook.*

Anne Thompson is a midwife educator, currently working with the Safe Motherhood Unit of the World Health Organization in Geneva. As Senior Lecturer at the Royal College of Midwives (UK) she helped set up the first UK MSc programme for Advanced Midwifery Practice with the University of Surrey. She has extensive work experience in Francophone Africa and recently has been Treasurer of the International Confederation of Midwives as well as a member of the UKCC Standards and Ethics Committee.

Delia Susana Veraguas Segura graduated as a *matrona* from the University of Chile in Valparaíso in 1971, and until the military coup in 1973 she worked in a neonatal unit in Valparaíso. In 1978 she also obtained a midwifery qualification in Britain. An experienced popular educator, she worked from 1981 to 1988 in the north of Nicaragua as a trainer of traditional midwives and as an administrator of the Casa de Preparación para el Parto Natural in Estelí. In 1993 she returned to Chile, where she works as a midwife in the primary health care sector in Viña del Mar, Chile.

Joan Walker is the Secretary General of the International Confederation of Midwives, and travels widely in this key co-ordinating role. She has many years of experience in midwifery practice and management in the UK. She was midwifery manager in a Health District Midwifery Service. She has also represented midwives at regional level at the Royal College of Midwives.

Foreword

About 10 years ago the world began to wake up to a 'forgotten tragedy' – the knowledge that at the end of the twentieth century women were still dying or having their lives permanently ruined by the simple, everyday experience of childbirth. The world – or at least, the industrialized world –learned with disbelief that there were places where women ran a risk of death in childbirth that was more than a hundred times that of their Western sisters.

The Safe Motherhood Initiative, launched with the support of WHO and many other agencies at the 1987 Nairobi Conference, challenged the world to halve the maternal mortality figures by the year 2000. WHO and the International Confederation of Midwives (ICM), together with UNICEF, picked up the challenge immediately, with a series of meetings focused on what midwives needed to do to bring their education and practice into line with the demands of safe motherhood programmes. The iniative was given new impetus in the World Summit for Children in 1990, the Cairo International Conference on Population and Development in 1994, and the Fourth International Women's Conference in Beijing in 1995. Also, by 1995, 90 of the 182 member states of WHO had some form of safe motherhood action plan. It was clear that in spite of the steadily worsening economic situation in the worst affected countries there was a very real commitment to action to save women's lives.

Lasting improvement in maternal health means involving much more than the health sector. Childbearing will only gradually become safe as women gain access to better education, better status, some economic independence, and a greater degree of control over their own reproductive lives. Universal access to essential services which are acceptable, appropriate, and welcoming, and improvements in the scope and quality of education for those who have the privilege of caring for childbearing women are essential goals. One of the strengths of this book is that it covers a wide range of issues which midwives must address if they are to meet the safe motherhood challenge effectively.

WHO's practical guide to safe motherhood programming, the Mother Baby Package, states:

> *The person best equipped to provide community-based, technologically appropriate and cost-effective care to women during their reproductive lives is the person with midwifery skills who lives in the community alongside the women she treats. Midwives understand women's concerns and preoccupations. They accompany women through their reproductive life-span, providing assistance at birth, then during adolescence, pregnancy and delivery. Most interventions related to the care of the mother and the newborn are within the capacity of the person with midwifery ...*

Midwives are often described as strong women, both individually and as a profession. It is probably truer to say that they are tenacious. What gives them strength, keeps them tenacious – and what shines through this book – is their conviction that childbearing women deserve a very special kind of service. This book is not just for midwives. It is for all decision makers, planners, campaigners, who work to make sure that each year fewer women die or are damaged in childbirth.

Dr Tomris Türmen
Executive Director, Family and Reproductive Health, WHO

Preface

These are exciting and thought provoking times. Midwifery internationally is in a state of flux. New developments affecting midwifery practice and research in developing and industrialised countries, have brought with them challenge and conflict. There are tensions between lay women's knowledge and power and medicalisation, between traditional caring functions and professionalisation, between individual care perspectives and public health perspectives, and between the need to provide services that are accessible and acceptable and the harsh economic realities of today's world. These themes run through many of the contributions to these two companion volumes, and the perspectives offered are rich and varied. Some chapters give an international overview of particular themes and are written by experts in those particular fields, others are written by experienced midwives and nurse-midwives who give concrete examples of the phenomena in question in a particular real life setting.

In the choice of contributors and themes I used as starting points the two major global initiatives that have most impacted on international midwifery practice in recent years, the Safe Motherhood Initiative and the Baby Friendly Hospital Initiative. With the edited contributions I have tried to bring together the theory and the practice of midwifery. I refer to these in their broadest sense: not only theoretical concepts in midwifery but theory about midwifery; not only clinical midwifery practice but the practice of midwifery policy and midwifery research. The books were written in the main by midwives themselves with their own profession in mind, but they also recognize the contribution that other disciplines, particularly the social sciences, can make to our understanding of what and who we are.

Much of the material in these volumes highlights the ways in which women across the world still lack power in relation to their own bodies, their own fertility and their own babies. Some of this powerlessness is the product of wider societal forces, of economic systems, of traditional beliefs, of modern commercial interests. Some of the responsibility, as many of the authors point out very clearly, also has to be laid directly at the door of the Western medical system and its advocates and implementers. Midwives must accept that we too have played our part in this. Our challenge now, as we approach the millennium, is to thoughtfully reconsider our role in the care of the health of women and their babies, and with this our role as women's advocates. Midwives have the potential of a unique and privileged relationship with women during important life events. This is something to be treasured. However, to my mind it is increasingly clear that we cannot confine our horizons to the provision of good individual care alone. Unique and privileged relationships bring with them wider social responsibilities and functions, to document, to research, to debate, to defend, and to advocate.

Susan F. Murray

Introduction

The first section of this volume (Chapters 1–4) concerns maternal health research in developing countries. It takes as a starting point some of the major direct causes of maternal mortality and morbidity in the world today. When the global Safe Motherhood Initiative was launched in 1987 by the World Health Organization (WHO), United Nations Family Planning Association (UNFPA), and the World Bank, it was in response to a growing awareness and concern about levels of maternal mortality and about the terrible disparity between rich and poor countries in this regard. Cross-country data revealed that there were five major direct obstetric causes of maternal death: haemorrhage, obstructed labour, sepsis, hypertensive diseases of pregnancy, and the complications of abortion. Midwives have increasingly become involved in research concerning safer motherhood issues, and the first four chapters are indicative of that involvement.

In Chapter 1 Barbara Kwast draws on her vast experience of work in Africa, Asia, and Latin America to consider the ways in which the death and disability caused by obstructed labour can be prevented. She reports findings from the major WHO study of the partograph, of which she was a principal co-ordinator, and discusses its relevance to the prevention of the complications of obstructed labour.

Susan Opoku describes in Chapter 2 the way in which maternal death from haemorrhage was investigated by a multidisciplinary team in Ghana, and how that research was used to design appropriate interventions.

The Safe Motherhood Initiative has highlighted the fact that it is not always enough just to provide health facilities and expect women to use them. In Chapter 3, Esnart Namakando examines what informs a woman's decision to use or not use existing maternity services, and provides a case study from Zambia. Susan Murray's review of the literature (Chapter 4) considers the impact of the introduction of user fees for maternity services. Economic reforms may be one of the principal developments of the 1990s that will militate against the work of the Safe Motherhood Initiative.

Section 2 (Chapters 5–7) considers some of the ways in which midwives' roles are expanding, or should be expanding, in response to our greater knowledge of women's reproductive health needs. Unwanted pregnancy is a major threat to women's health and women's lives in much of the world, most particularly in countries where abortion is illegal or difficult to obtain. In Chapter 5, Charlotte Hord and Grace Delano highlight this tragedy and discuss how midwives can be involved in life-saving treatment and in service provision, using specific country examples. In Chapter 6, Patricia Semeraro takes up the theme of appropriate postpartum contraceptive services and considers the role of the midwife within these. Then, in Chapter 7, Susan Murray and Delia Susana Veraguas give a portrait of one way in which the midwife's role may be extended. The university-trained Chilean midwife, the *matrona*, is the health professional in the public sector who provides reproductive health care to women throughout most of their life span, from adolescence through to the menopause.

Section 3 (Chapters 8–11) deals with some midwifery education and training issues of particular relevance to developing countries. Since Deborah Maine questioned the effectiveness of traditional birth attendant (TBA) training in her highly influential document, *Safe Motherhood Programs: Options and Issues* (Columbia University, 1990), debates have raged over the value of training traditional midwives at all. In Chapter 8, Maureen Minden and Marta Levitt, both experienced TBA trainers, take issue with those who consider the role of traditional midwives only in terms of their capacity to carry out 'essential obstetric functions'. They argue that the emphasis on the prevention of direct obstetric death was a by-product of the need to identify clearly definable indicators as a basis for launching and promoting the Safe Motherhood Initiative. There is nothing quite as finite as death, and it was graphic images, such as that used by Malcolm Potts of a jumbo jet filled with women crashing every 4 hours, that galvanized governments and aid agencies into action. Where such indicators become problematic is when they confine how we see the solution. Levitt and Minden characterize the current debate as one between a 'Crisis Management Perspective' and a 'Community Development Perspective', and outline the assumptions behind these opposing positions.

The third section of the book concerns the ways in which midwifery education can creatively respond to the increased awareness of maternal mortality and morbidity issues in developing countries. In Chapter 9, Gloria Betts, an experienced midwifery teacher from West Africa, gives her views on the midwifery education needs of the future, and her personal vision of the kind of midwife who will be required to meet the challenges of midwifery practice at community, first referral, regional, and national level. In Chapter 10, Lola Payne gives a concrete example from MotherCare Nigeria of what can be achieved when in-service training is used to extend midwives' roles by improving their ability to provide both good technical care (life-saving skills) and psychological care (interpersonal communication skills). Chapter 11 takes a challenging look at the importance and meaning of supervision in midwifery. Marie-Claude Foster offers a dynamic and reflective model which is based on an understanding of 'midwifery as artistry'.

The final section of this volume (Chapters 12 and 13) looks at midwifery internationally with two fascinating contributions. In Chapter 12, Joan Walker and Anne Thompson give us a detailed account of the history of the International Confederation of Midwives, and of its significant current-day role in the promotion of safer motherhood. The final chapter provides us with an overview of some of the influences on the status of midwives in different countries, and how these affect their practice. Raymond DeVries, a sociologist, suggests that, to fully understand the effectiveness of midwifery care, we also need to know how midwifery fits into that particular society. While midwives across the world share the common tasks of assisting at birth and caring for the health of women, they do not share a common status. In giving us an overview of the diversity across cultures, of the impact of technology and of conceptualisations of risk, he ties together issues raised in many of the preceding contributions, and offers important insights for the effective implementation of midwifery programmes.

Acknowledgements

I wish to express my warm thanks to the many people who contributed to these two volumes of International Perspectives on Midwifery. Much labour went into these pages, and I know that for many of the authors this was done a little wearily, at the end of long working days, or nights, full of other priorities and commitments, and at the mercy of erratic power supplies and unreliable postal services.

I would particularly like to thank Helen Armstrong, Gabrielle Palmer, Barbara Kwast and Joan Walker for their invaluable initial suggestions on contributors. I also wish to thank Fiona Watson whose incisive assistance in editing at a crucial moment helped to save the books from foundering, and Della R. Sherratt, Head of Overseas Education Developments, Avon and Gloucester College of Health, whose comments as the publisher's referee were immensely valuable.

Dedication

The women whose deaths make up the maternal mortality statistics are daughters, sisters, wives, lovers, and mothers. Their loss is deeply felt by those around them. This volume is dedicated to the memory of one such woman, Rosa Lopez Araos, and to the future of her granddaughters Kerry, Francesca, and Elisabeth, who never had the chance to know her.

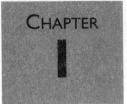

CHAPTER

1

Prolonged and Obstructed Labour in Developing Countries: Steps to Reduce a Neglected Tragedy

Barbara E. Kwast

In this chapter we consider in detail the research evidence concerning one of the major causes of maternal death and morbidity in developing countries. First, the devastating effects of prolonged and obstructed labour are reviewed, and the effectiveness of the commonly available screening processes is considered. The importance of community outreach and education is highlighted. Then, the role of the partograph in monitoring and preventing complications is discussed, as are the results of the World Health Organization (WHO) multicentre trial of the partograph carried out in Indonesia, Malaysia, and Thailand. Finally, the necessary clinical diagnosis and management of obstructed labour are outlined for when it does occur.

MORTALITY AND MORBIDITY CAUSED BY OBSTRUCTED LABOUR

The journey of the baby through the birth canal during labour and delivery is the most dangerous time for both mother and infant. The lethal triad of haemorrhage, sepsis, and obstructed labour causes the majority of deaths during labour and the first day postpartum. Women may be left with disabling conditions, such as severe anaemia, infertility, or vesicovaginal fistula, while new-borns could be damaged by asphyxia or cerebral palsy. The case history of Rachel (see box on page 2) illustrates the medical, socioeconomic, and cultural factors which can have devastating consequences in labour and delivery.

Obstructed labour is caused by mechanical failures and not by disturbances of uterine physiology. The fetus fails to descend into the birth canal in spite of good uterine contractions and labour is obstructed when further progress is impossible without assistance (Lawson, 1967). Three-quarters of all maternal deaths (378,250 per year) are due to 'direct' causes: haemorrhage, sepsis, abortion, eclampsia, and

Rachel

Rachel was 13 years old when she married a farmer who had no formal education. The family lived in a remote village in grain-producing temperate highlands. They owned a bull and had a small home with no electricity. Rachel's first child was born dead in hospital, after 4 days in labour at home. The obstructed labour resulted in a vesico-vaginal fistula which was repaired in a specialized hospital. Rachel was instructed to come to the hospital during her next pregnancy after the eighth month. Rachel became pregnant 3 years after the fistula surgery, with a much-wanted child. She lived far from the health centre and received no antenatal care. At 7 months, she started to bleed from the genital tract after fetching water from the river. Labour started immediately and the membranes ruptured. Rachel was taken to the hospital, after she had been in labour for 3 days at home. She was in severe distress with a high temperature and rapid pulse. Although the baby was small, birth could not progress because of scar tissue from the earlier surgery. The baby was dead on admission and, according to Rachel, she had not felt fetal movements for 1 month. The baby was delivered by destructive operation vaginally. Rachel had pneumonia and severe puerperal sepsis. As her condition worsened, she had an emergency laparotomy followed by a hysterectomy because of extensive septic necrosis of a ruptured uterus. She went into renal failure and her condition became critical. In spite of blood transfusions, renal dialysis, and aggressive antibiotic therapy, she died 27 days after the birth of her dead premature infant.

obstructed labour and/or ruptured uterus. Data from 11 population-based studies show that 11% of these deaths are due to obstructed labour (including death from ruptured uterus) (Maine, 1991), which is equivalent to 41,607 maternal deaths per year or one death every 13 minutes. A further 28% of deaths are due to haemorrhage and another 11% to sepsis, many of which are also due to prolonged and obstructed labour that could be avoided.

Figure 1.1 presents detailed data from community-based studies on the percentage of maternal deaths due to obstructed labour and/or ruptured uterus, haemorrhage, and sepsis. Data from community-based studies are rare because such studies are expensive and difficult to undertake. Furthermore, definitions remain problematic. Deaths from ruptured uterus are usually preceded by obstructed labour, but may be classified as haemorrhage. Likewise, deaths from obstructed labour may be classified as due to puerperal sepsis.

There is a paucity of data on prolonged labour, but two studies conducted in Indonesia and Guatemala found that the incidence of prolonged labour was 4.8% (Alisjahbana *et al.*, 1995) and 2.8% (Schieber and Szasdi, 1994), respectively. Prolonged labour was defined in these studies as 'hard labour' (in which normal activity is no longer possible) lasting longer than 12 h. There was no validation against medical records in either study and the data need to be interpreted with caution.

Region, country, area	Date	Obstructed labour (%)	Ruptured uterus (%)	Haemorrhage (postpartum) (%)	Puerperal sepsis (%)	Reference
Africa						
Ethiopia						
Addis Ababa	1981–1983	–	8.3 [4.4][a]	12.5 [6.7][a]	4.2 [2.2][a]	Kwast (1988)
Egypt						
Giza	1985–1986	8.3	–	38	11	Kane et al. (1992)
Assiut	1987	–	13.8	24.1	6.9	Abdullah et al. (1992)
Asia						
Bangladesh						
Tangail	1983–1984	21[b]		17	10	Alauddin (1986)
Jamalpur	1980–1982	20[b]		12	12	Khan (1986)
Matlab	1974–1976	9[b]		22	3	Lindpainter (1982)
Papua New Guinea	1976–1983	11[b]		33	31	Mola and Aitkin (1984)
India						
Andra Pradesh	1984–1985	–	7.9 [5.3][a]	9.4 [6.3][a]	33.2 [22.2][a]	Bhatia (1993)
North India	1985–1986	11.8 [7.3][a]	–	29.4 [18.5][a]	26.4 [16.4][a]	Kumar et al. (1989)

[a] In brackets = Percentage of both direct and indirect deaths.
[b] Percentage for obstructed labour and ruptured uterus.

Figure 1.1 Maternal deaths from obstructed labour, ruptured uterus, haemorrhage, and puerperal sepsis (as percentage of direct obstetric causes), community-based studies.

There are also few studies on referral patterns for prolonged or obstructed labour. In a rural area of Guatemala, 18.9% of referrals from traditional birth attendants (TBAs) were for prolonged labour (O'Rourke, 1995), and in southern Tanzania 82.4% of referrals were due to obstructed or prolonged labour, with 50% of these diagnosed as having a ruptured uterus (Urrio, 1991). The WHO multicentre trial in eight hospitals in Indonesia, Malaysia, and Thailand reported a pre-intervention incidence of prolonged labour (>18 h) of 6.4% (WHO, 1994a).

Complications as a result of obstructed labour

Figure 1.2 shows an incidence of obstructed labour of up to 20% in specific hospital studies in Africa and Asia. In eastern Nigeria, 73% of obstetric hysterectomies were performed for ruptured uterus after obstructed labour (Osefo, 1989). In the same city, Enugu, another study reported that the leading complications from obstructed labour were puerperal sepsis (57%), postpartum haemorrhage (15%), ruptured uterus (14%), and genital lacerations (14%) (Ozumba and Uchegbu, 1991). Recent data from Ibadan show similar proportions, with the additional complications of pre-

Region and country	Date	Cases of obstructed labour	Percentage of deliveries	References
Africa				
Ethiopia	1990	143	18.0	Kelly (1992)
Nigeria	1985–1989	527	4.7	Ozumba et al. (1991)
Zaire	1984–1986	740	19.9	FHI[a] (1988)
Zaire	1981–1982	319	17.8	Janowitz et al. (1984)
Asia				
Bangladesh	1976–1980	1494	10.2	Begum et al. (1981)
Bangladesh	1979–1980	1494	11.5	Bhuiyan et al. (1981)
India	1977	128	2.9	Basu (1977)

[a] Family Health International

Figure 1.2 Prevalence of obstructed labour, hospital studies.

eclampsia (14.7%) and eclampsia (4.2%) which can develop acutely in the process of obstructed labour (Konje et al., 1992).

Uterine rupture is a disastrous complication of labour and delivery, showing rates as high as 11/1000 deliveries in hospitals in Africa, with mortality ranging from 9 to 42%. While most uterine ruptures are caused by obstructed labour, 20–25% of ruptures are due to a previous caesarean scar and 3–22% are caused by inappropriate interventions by health workers or TBAs (Liskin, 1992). A review of the literature from the past three decades indicates that the incidence of ruptured uterus in hospital has not declined, and an increase of 1/702 deliveries in 1978 to 1/500 deliveries in 1987 was reported from eastern Nigeria. Case fatality dropped from 43% to 15% in the same period (Iloabachie and Agwu, 1990). A decline in mortality from ruptured uterus in hospitals has also been reported from Guinea and South Africa (Balde and Bastert, 1990; Lachman et al., 1985). This decline has been attributed to improvements in obstetric care and the use of the partograph, together with improved access to maternity services.

Perinatal mortality as a result of obstructed labour

Fetal loss caused by obstructed labour and ruptured uterus is enormous. WHO estimates that some 3% of new-born babies (3.6 million) suffer moderate or severe birth asphyxia following obstructed labour. Of these, about 840,000 die and an equal number suffer brain damage that leads to cerebral palsy, seizures, and other handicaps, including learning disorders (WHO, 1993b). Almost all women with a ruptured uterus are delivered of a dead fetus. In eastern Nigeria, for example, perinatal mortality in obstructed labour was 294/1000 births compared with 47/1000 for all hospital deliveries (Ozumba and Uchegbu, 1991). The early perinatal mortality rates (EPMRs) in a rural district hospital in Kenya for prolonged labour (>18 h), obstructed labour, and ruptured uterus were 177/1000, 428/1000, and 940/1000 total births, respectively (Kavoo-Linge and Rogo, 1992). Of fistula patients in Ethiopia, 92.7% had a still birth (Kelly and Kwast, 1993).

Sequelae of obstructed labour

The most disabling and humiliating consequence of obstructed labour is obstetric fistula. The true incidence of vesicovaginal fistula (VVF) is not known, but it is common in certain well-defined geographic areas in sub-Saharan Africa, stretching from Nigeria in the west to Ethiopia and Somalia in the east, and in parts of the Asian subcontinent (WHO, 1989). About 25% of women with a VVF also develop a rectovaginal fistula. A detailed study of fistulas in Ethiopia showed that 97% were due to prolonged and/or obstructed labour, with a mean duration of 3.9 days. Such damage is only reversible at great cost or not reversible at all. Of these women, 52.3% were left by their husbands following the fistula. This devastating situation for thousands of women only a few years away from the turn of the twentieth century is witness to the dismal failure of maternity services to reach women in their most critical hours of child-bearing.

Factors contributing to prevalence of obstructed labour

MEDICAL FACTORS

Cephalopelvic disproportion (CPD) is the most common cause of obstructed labour. It is often due to general pelvic contraction or pelvic deformity because of rickets or osteomalacia. Women's reproductive health is thus intimately related to their nutritional status. In developing countries, 450 million adult women, mainly in South Asia and sub-Saharan Africa, are estimated to be stunted as a result of childhood protein-energy malnutrition. Early child-bearing, before growth of the pelvis is complete, is another reason for CPD. Births to adolescents currently represent 15–20% of all births in the 11 African countries for which current data are available (Center for Population Options, 1992).

Other important causes of CPD are malpresentation or malposition of the fetus, impacted shoulders after delivery of the head, abnormalities of the vagina and perineum due to previous scarring from surgery, use of traditional medicines which have oxytocic properties, female genital mutilation, and tumours of the uterus or ovaries.

CULTURAL FACTORS

A spontaneous delivery at home is the most-valued achievement of a successful pregnancy (Public Opinion Polls, 1993). Women may feel that they lose status in society when they deliver in hospital, as this is a less courageous way to give birth. When labour results in an operative delivery, a sense of reproductive failure may be experienced. These feelings may deter women who have had a caesarean section from using hospitals at subsequent deliveries.

HEALTH SERVICE FACTORS

Estimates for 1993 show that only 59% of pregnant women receive antenatal care in the developing world; 37% of births occur in institutions; and 55% have a trained birth attendant at delivery (WHO, 1993b). A number of maternal death audits in hospitals during the past decade have revealed that in 80–90% of cases avoidable factors, such as shortage or non-availability of personnel, equipment, drugs, blood for transfusion, and functioning operating theatres to deal with emergencies, were present (Kwast, 1992). A study in India found that inadequate medical treatment contributed to 36–47% of maternal deaths in hospitals (Pillai, 1993). In southern Tanzania, maternal deaths following dystocia or prolonged labour in hospitals with a low rate of partograph use were twice those in hospitals with a 50% use (Price, 1984). Staff factors, errors of judgement, lack of expertise, and omission of essential tasks contributed to 10% of mortality. Of maternal deaths outside the hospital, 64% were due to failure to act on risk factors at the village (38%), health centre (15%), or dispensary (11%) (Price, 1984). Delay in referral and transportation accounted for a further 15% of deaths.

PREVENTION OF DEATH AND MORBIDITY FROM OBSTRUCTED LABOUR

Obstructed labour in developed countries has been virtually eradicated during the past five decades. Improvements in the standard of living, increased access to maternity services, availability of antibiotics and blood transfusion, and improved techniques in surgery and anaesthesia are responsible for this.

Not all deliveries have to take place in hospital. If there are well-trained professional midwives available to conduct home births, efficient referral systems, and hospitals equipped to deal with emergencies, obstructed labour may be prevented outside the hospital.

The key to prevention of obstructed labour lies in good-quality, continuous obstetric care. While maternal mortality is lower in women who receive antenatal care compared to those who do not, alone it does not guarantee a safe birth. Antenatal care, care in labour and delivery, postpartum and neonatal care, and family planning all require attention and active community involvement to ensure a reduction in incidence of obstructed labour.

Antenatal assessment for predictors of obstructed labour

Unfortunately, there are no risk screening tools that can predict which women will develop complications during labour. No single measurement can diagnose CPD during the antenatal period. Past obstetric history, patient's height, and abdominal and pelvic assessment all need to be considered.

Summary of antenatal assessment for predictors of obstructed labour
- At every antenatal contact discuss the recommended place for delivery when an abnormality or complication is detected.
- Try to speak with the partner and/or relatives to encourage preparation for institutional delivery if complications are detected during pregnancy.
- Encourage any primigravida ≤17 years and ≤1.50 m to deliver in a health centre under the supervision of a midwife or in a hospital.
- Inform women and their family of any malpresentation at term and encourage delivery in a health facility.
- Women with previous caesarean section or previous traumatic vaginal delivery should be counselled, together with a family member, about the desirability of a hospital delivery.

PAST OBSTETRIC HISTORY

Previous operative delivery, perinatal death, and birth weight data provide some indication of pelvic size. In Zaire, women with a poor obstetric history were 10 times more likely to have an obstructed labour than women with a good obstetric history (Maine, 1991). However, only 10% of women with a poor obstetric history experienced obstructed labour. Thus, obstetric history alone is not a sensitive indicator of risk of obstructed labour.

PATIENT'S HEIGHT

Studies in Mozambique, Sierra Leone, and Tanzania report that low maternal height is associated significantly with interventions during labour (Aitken and Walls, 1986; Roosmalen and Brand, 1992; Liljestrand et al., 1991). Philpott's (1982) study of Shona and Zulu women found some association between short stature and CPD, but that the range was too wide to be used for screening purposes. This also applied to foot measurements. A sensitive cut-off level for height to use in the prediction of CPD can only be developed by community surveys for height measurement. Current evidence suggests the cut-off point is ≤1.45 m for Asia (WHO, 1994b).

ABDOMINAL AND PELVIC ASSESSMENT

Midwives trained with Western textbooks learn that "in primigravidae the fetal head is normally engaged at 38–40 weeks of pregnancy". This is misleading because in African women engagement of the head in the primipara usually does not happen until the active phase of labour (±3 cm dilatation) and in the multipara not until the late active phase of labour (6–7 cm dilatation). It is generally thought that this is because of a high angle of pelvic inclination in African women.

A head-fitting test is usually difficult to perform, but a negative result may be due to factors other than CPD (Philpott, 1982). If pelvic assessment is to be attempted it should not be carried out before 38 weeks of pregnancy. It is not an easy procedure, but midwives should be taught how to measure the diagonal conjugate of the brim of the pelvis. External pelvic measurements are virtually useless (Lawson, 1967). If a pregnant woman has a severely deformed pelvis such that she needs an elective caesarean section, this will become evident from clinical assessment. If there is a suspicion of CPD, primigravidae should have a carefully controlled trial of labour, even in the absence of any other abnormalities or complications.

Screening for risk of obstructed labour should be carried out during the last 2 weeks of pregnancy, at the onset of labour, and during the process of labour. In the antenatal period, an abdominal examination should be conducted in order to detect an abnormally large fetus, a persistent transverse lie, or a multiple pregnancy.

Community outreach

A study of TBA referrals to hospital in Guatemala showed a high sensitivity (78%) for accuracy of detection of malpresentations, among both trained and untrained TBAs. This potential needs to be strengthened wherever TBAs practice. Analysis of data from the demographic and health surveys shows that although antenatal care may be predominantly carried out by physicians and professional midwives, there is a shift over to TBAs for care at delivery (Kwast, 1993). The actual degree of the involvement of the TBA varies according to the setting; in some areas it is the custom that the TBA be called only after labour to tie the baby's cord and to remove the placenta. In the Bolivian Andes mountains, husbands assist at their wives' deliveries, and it is they who need to be involved in learning about complications.

It is vital that the formal health care system makes itself familiar with the customs and traditions of the communities it serves, and that antenatal care interventions are linked to delivery care. Decision-making structures also have to be recognized and worked with. It is often mothers-in-law and husbands, together with traditional healers, who decide about referral to hospital care. The pregnant woman herself may be relatively powerless. In such a situation, just teaching women in antenatal clinics about danger signs is unlikely to have much impact. Antenatal care needs to be far more of a community outreach activity than it is at present. The hospital staff need to work to build up trust, and at village level the midwife needs to foster a dialogue with TBAs and with families to expedite delivery in a health facility when complications are detected. Community awareness (male and female) of the dangers of prolonged labour can be fostered using methods such as picture brochures, radio spots, and audiovisuals designed with community help (MotherCare, 1994). It is my experience that men on every continent want to know about the conditions that may constitute risks to their wives during pregnancy. The barrier to communication often lies in the attitude or the fears of the service providers.

Mechanisms must be created to get services closer to women or women closer to services when complications arise (WHO, 1991). The success stories have been programmes that combined community development activities, community-based antenatal care, establishment of mothers' waiting homes or prayer houses on the rural hospital grounds, and efficient in-patient obstetric services (Brennan and Umoh, 1993; Poovan et al., 1990).

The early detection of complications during labour

Many women in developing countries do not have access to health facilities for economic, geographical, or cultural reasons. Who, then, should undertake screening at home to detect complications which have not been diagnosed during the antenatal period and who should supervise child-bearing and diagnose abnormal progress in labour?

AT VILLAGE LEVEL

Where husbands or other family members assist at deliveries, they need to be instructed about complications. Where there is a TBA, she should be taught to recognize, through abdominal examination, both large babies presenting by the vertex and malpresentations. In every village, at least one house in a cluster should have 1.50 m marked off on a door-post as a yardstick for very small women. With a little ingenuity, and community consultation, it may be possible to agree on time periods, such as sunset to sunrise (12 h) or the number of prayer calls from a mosque (two or three), beyond which a woman should not be kept in labour in the village. However, we have to recognize that the definition of labour is as difficult for women as it is for the medical profession, added to which there may be cultural values by which women go through labour alone and in silence. It may also take several hours before arrangements can be made to transport a woman to a health facility.

AT A HEALTH POST, PRIVATE MATERNITY CLINIC, OR HEALTH CENTRE

A trained midwife may be practising at the village, in the health post, or at the health centre. In a well-functioning maternity service she will act as the back-up for the TBA in the village. She will be the link between the TBA and the hospital and be connected, hopefully with transport, to a referral hospital. A serious commitment to the reduction of maternal deaths will require the delegation of some essential obstetric functions to such midwives in the periphery, who must be trained adequately, equipped with the appropriate technology, and then be supported by physicians in the referral facility. It is recommended that all midwives practising at this level use the partograph to monitor labour.

THE ROLE OF THE PARTOGRAPH IN DEVELOPING COUNTRIES

The WHO partograph

The pattern of progressive cervical dilatation in normal labour was identified by Friedman over 40 years ago (Friedman, 1955). The application of this knowledge to the management of labour with the aid of a partograph to record the progress of labour graphically was developed by Philpott and Castle (1972a, 1972b) in Zimbabwe, Studd (1973) in the United Kingdom, and O'Driscoll (1973) in Ireland, all of whom reported improved results in the outcome of labour.

The WHO partograph (*Figure 1.3*) closely resembles that promoted by Philpott in Zimbabwe in the 1970s. The central feature is the cervicograph, where cervical dilatation is plotted against time. While accepting that the transition from the latent to the active phase of labour may take place at differing cervical dilatations in individual cases, 3 cm dilatation is the most frequent at which the transition takes place, so the cervicograph is marked accordingly. In the active phase of labour, a rate of dilatation of 1 cm/h represents the mean dilatation rate of the slowest 10% of Zimbabwe primigravidae, and all partographs assume 1 cm/h or faster as an acceptable level of dilatation. This rate is designated the *alert line* on the partograph. When cervical dilatation strays to the right of the alert line, women in labour at centres without facilities for caesarean section should be transferred to a centre where such facilities exist.

The *action line* on the partograph is drawn parallel to, but 4 h to the right of, the alert line. When cervical dilatation reaches this line, labour progress is dangerously slow and obstetric decisions concerning management are essential. The '4 h action line' was found by Philpott and Bird (Philpott and Castle, 1972b; Bird, 1978) to be the most efficient means of identifying particularly slow labours and so avoiding unnecessarily early or dangerously late intervention.

These cervicographic features are incorporated into the WHO partograph, together with the facility to record all other essential observations in labour on an hourly or half-hourly basis. Experience with partography has shown that fewer recording errors are made when the action, alert, and latent phase lines are pre-printed on the partograph, rather than drawn by the observer. When women are admitted in the active phase of labour, recordings are plotted directly onto the appropriate part of the active phase, with the admission dilatation being placed *on* the alert line. If the woman is admitted in the latent phase, recordings are plotted at the beginning of the cervicograph at 0 h. Observations made on women who progress from the latent to the active phase within 8 h are transferred to the appropriate part

9

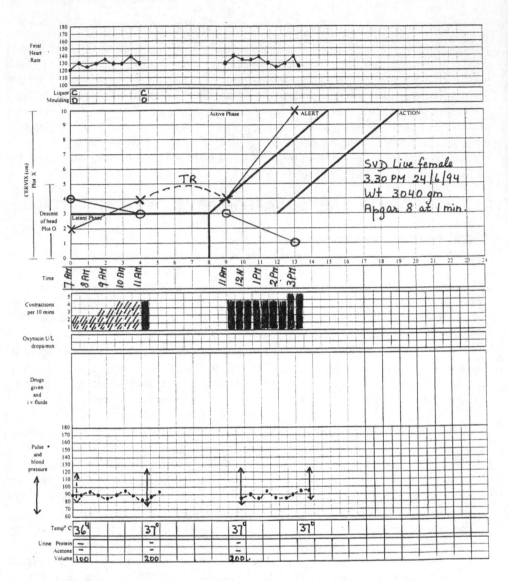

Figure 1.3 The WHO partograph. The maternal and fetal condition together with the progress of labour is recorded on the graph against the passage of time. This figure shows a woman admitted in the latent phase of labour at 7 a.m. with 2 cm dilatation; her recordings started at the beginning of the graph. The head is four-fifths above the inlet of the pelvis and contractions are two in 10 minutes, lasting between 20 and 40 seconds. At 11 a.m., 4 hours after admission, the cervical dilatation was 4 cm and the woman in the active phase of the first stage of labour. The dilatation is now transferred *onto* the alert line because this line represents the progress of 1 cm/hour in the active phase (the lower limit of normal progress). The head is three-fifths above the inlet. All other fetal and maternal observations are also transferred. The contractions at 11 a.m. are four in 10 minutes, lasting more than 40 seconds. At 3 p.m. the cervix is fully dilated (10 cm), the head is one-fifth above the brim, the contractions are five in 10 minutes, lasting more than 40 seconds. The woman has a spontaneous vertex delivery 10 minutes later, of a female child with an Agpar score of eight at 1 minute.

Criteria for commencing a partograph

In latent phase (cervix 0–2 cm)
Contractions: two or more in 10 minutes, lasting 20 seconds or more.
In active phase (cervix ≥3 cm)
Contractions: one or more in 10 minutes, lasting 20 seconds or more.

of the partograph, placing the first cervical dilatation recorded at 3 cm or more at the appropriate place on the alert line.

Vaginal examinations to assess cervical dilatation are the key element of partographic observations and labour management, so are normally made every 4 h. Other observations are made and recorded at conventional intervals. As an observational tool, the method is economical and efficient; it obviates the need for additional writing, except in unusual cases. The descent of the head is assessed in fifths above the brim (inlet) of the pelvis and the recording is made on the cervicograph (see *Figure 1.3* and WHO, 1993a). Contractions are timed for length and frequency and the appropriate number of boxes shaded, according to a key that indicates the duration, in the space provided below that cervicograph. The partograph provides spaces for all maternal and fetal observations.

It has proved crucial to establish criteria (see box above) for starting a partograph to ensure that one is not begun for women not actually in labour.

WHO organized a multicentre trial on the use of the partograph in the management of labour in eight hospitals in Indonesia, Malaysia, and Thailand for 15 months from January 1990 (WHO, 1994a, 1994b).

While the efficacy of the partograph was well described by Philpott, O'Driscoll, and Studd in the early 1970s, there had been a paucity of publications for two decades. WHO needed up-to-date research to promote this tool universally as part of the Safe Motherhood Initiative. As the strategy for implementation of the partograph begins in the referral hospital, the WHO study was carried out at hospital level. However, implementation and operations research is still advocated in peripheral centres to demonstrate the efficacy of the partograph as a referral tool.

Results of the WHO multicentre trial of the partograph

A total of 35,484 women were included in the study, of whom 93% had visited an antenatal clinic at least twice; most deliveries were planned in the eight participating hospitals. There were 39.1% nullipara, 51.9% multipara (1–4), and 8.9% grand multipara (5+), with a mean age of 27 years, mean maternal height of 1.53 m, mean gestational age of 39 weeks, and mean birth weights for singletons of 3065 g and for multiple births of 2276 g. Of the women admitted, 25% were in the latent phase of labour, 62% had 3–9 cm dilatation, and 13% were in the second stage of labour. Spontaneous labour occurred in 85.6% of the women, and 7.1% were induced. The total caesarean section rate was 12.1% (2.5% elective and 9.5% emergency) and the operative vaginal delivery rate was 9.9%. Neonatal deaths were under-recorded, but the stillborn rate was 2.6%. In most of these cases the fetus was already dead *in utero*

Protocol for labour management with the WHO partograph

MANAGEMENT OF NORMAL LATENT AND ACTIVE PHASES
1. Do not augment or intervene unless complications develop.
2. Artificial rupture of membranes (ARM):
   •active phase – at any time.
   •latent phase – no ARM.

MANAGEMENT OF LABOUR BETWEEN ALERT AND ACTION LINES
1. Do not intervene or augment labour with oxytocin unless complications develop (oxytocin augmentation should never be given in a maternity or health centre without facilities for operative delivery).
2. ARM at first vaginal examination between alert and action line, if still intact.
3. If in a peripheral unit, transfer patient, unless delivery is imminent or labour progresses very well when membranes have just been ruptured at first vaginal examination between alert and action line.

MANAGEMENT OF LABOUR AT OR BEYOND ACTION LINE
1. Full medical assessment. Patient should now be in hospital. If still in peripheral clinic, urgent transfer to hospital is required.
2. Consider intravenous (IV) infusion and/or bladder catheterization and/or analgesia.
3. Options:
   •Delivery (normally caesarean section) if fetal distress or obstructed labour.
   •Oxytocin augmentation through IV infusion, if no contraindications.
   •Conservative management – supportive therapy only.
   •Further review (in cases continuing in labour):
      1. Vaginal examination after 3 h, then after a further 2 h, and again after a further 2 h. Progress <1 cm/h between any of these examinations means delivery is indicated.
      2. Fetal heart while on oxytocin must be checked at least every half hour.

TIMING OF OBSERVATIONS IN THE NORMAL LATENT PHASE

	Ideal	Minimum acceptable
Vaginal examination	4 h	8 h
Descent of head	4 h	8 h
Contractions	0.5 h	4 h
Fetal heart	0.5 h	4 h
Temperature, pulse, and blood pressure, urine	4 h	4 h

(cont.)

Protocol for labour management with the WHO partograph (cont.)

TIMING OF OBSERVATIONS IN THE NORMAL ACTIVE PHASE (UP TO THE ACTION LINE)

	Ideal	Minimum acceptable
Vaginal examination	4 h	4 h
Descent of head	4 h	4 h
Contractions	0.5 h	2 h
Fetal heart	0.5 h	I h
Temperature, pulse, and blood pressure	4 h	4 h

Vaginal examination should, as a rule, be restricted to 4 h intervals, but may be carried out more frequently in the advanced first stage when delivery is expected within 4 h (7 cm or more) or if problems develop.

---

on admission. There were 47 maternal deaths and 55 women with ruptured uterus, the majority of whom had been admitted to the hospital in neglected obstructed labour; this illustrates the dilemma that partography only influences labour outcome if women are cared for by a trained attendant who can read and perform accurate observations in labour.

Labour outcome was related to maternal age and parity. A steady decline in obstetric performance was found with advancing years and increasing parity, resulting in an increase in caesarean sections and still births. The outcome of teenage pregnancy was excellent. The only association between labour outcome and small maternal stature was an increased caesarean section rate, although even among very short women (<140 cm), only 32% were delivered abdominally.

Although these hospital patients were not representative of the population as a whole, the pelvic capacity in the Asian teenage women was clearly different from that in their sisters in Africa.

The results confirmed recommendations (Prendiville et al., 1988; Elbourne et al., 1988) that the optimum management of the third stage of labour is to administer intramuscular Syntometrine after delivery of the head, followed by controlled cord-traction delivery of the placenta. The incidence of postpartum haemorrhage (PPH) fell with increasing parity, confirming the findings of other recent studies of higher levels of PPH among nullipara and low rates among grand multipara (Gilbert et al., 1987; Combs et al., 1992; Eidelman et al., 1988).

OUTCOME OF LABOUR

The most striking effect of introducing the partograph was that the number of labours augmented with oxytocin fell from 20.7% to 9.1% (*Figure 1.4*). Despite this, the mean duration of observed labour after admission fell from 5.72 to 5.05 h, with an increase in short labours of less than 12 h and a reduction of almost 50% in the proportion of prolonged labours (>18 h), from 6.4% to 3.4%. Vaginal examinations in labour fell from a mean of 1.78 per woman to 1.52. The mean period for oxytocin use in

	Before partograph (%)	After partograph (%)
Total deliveries	18,254 (100)	17,230 (100)
Labour >18 h	1147 (6.4)	589 (3.4)[1]
Labour augmented	3785 (20.7)	1573 (9.1)[2]
Delivery (singletons only)		
Spontaneous cephalic	13,186 (72.4)	12,704 (73.9)
Vaginal breech	618 (3.4)	591 (3.4)
Vacuum/forceps	1793 (9.8)	1649 (9.6)
Emergency caesarean section	1802 (9.9)	1495 (8.7)
Postpartum haemorrhage	1710 (9.4)	1510 (8.8)
Postpartum sepsis	127 (0.7)	37 (0.2)[3]
Intrapartum still birth	92 (0.5)	55 (0.3)
Neonatal admissions to intensive/ special care	2061 (11.2)	1684 (9.6)

Slight discrepancies in numbers and percentages are due to missing or incomplete data.
[1] $p = 0.002$.   [2] $p = 0.023$.   [3] $p = 0.028$.

Figure 1.4 Outcome of labour before and after introduction of the WHO partograph.

augmented labours increased from 3.83 to 4.34 h, probably because of a better selection of women who needed this intervention. Postpartum sepsis fell, especially among women who had undergone caesarean sections. With regard to neonatal outcome, a significant improvement was achieved in reducing intrapartum still births.

CERVICAL DILATATION RATES
The rates of dilatation in labour of a subgroup of women defined as 'normal' were studied in detail. 'Normal' women were defined as those for whom no complications had been identified prior to labour, and in whom the baby presented by the vertex and was alive at the onset of spontaneous labour at term. Among these 17,875 women, the mean rate of cervical dilatation (regardless of the admission dilatation) was 2.87 cm/h. The rate for nullipara was 1.63 cm/h, for multipara 3.69 cm/h, and for grand multipara (5+) 4.14 cm/h. The mean rate was close to 1 cm/h in the latent phase and >2 cm/h in the active phase. The slowest 25% of women dilated at a mean rate just over 1 cm/h, with the slowest 10% just under 1 cm/h.

These findings provide a guide for midwives as to the speed with which labour can progress and encourage preparedness for delivery at different stages of admission dilatations. They also provide information on how quickly a multipara can obstruct in labour. With these parameters in use, and the intelligent interpretation of the progress of labour and when to seek medical help, it is unacceptable for a patient to be in prolonged or obstructed labour in a maternity unit where the midwife is in charge.

PROGRESS OF LABOUR RELATIVE TO THE ALERT AND ACTION LINES
There were 8810 'normal' women in the study whose labour was managed using a partograph. Of these, 73% were admitted in the active phase of labour and 27% in

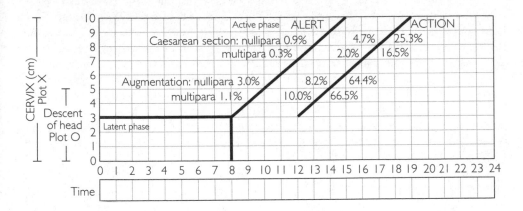

Figure 1.5 Caesarean section and augmentation rates by parity and course of labour for all normal women with an active phase.

the latent phase. Only nine women were delivered within the latent phase (<8 h) by caesarean section. Note that only 112 women (1.3% of the total) failed to progress to the active phase within 8 h of admission. The majority of latent-phase admissions were nulliparous women, and their subsequent course of labour was longer compared to women who were admitted in the active phase.

Of the 8698 women with an active phase of labour, 73% remained on or left of the alert line. Of the 27% who moved to the right of the alert line, 864 (10% of the total) reached the action line.

THE 'TRANSFER ZONE' – BETWEEN ALERT AND ACTION LINE

According to the management protocol for the partograph, women whose dilatation moves to the 'transfer zone', the area between the alert and action lines, should be referred. *Figure 1.5* clearly shows that intervention rates increased as labour progress deviated to the right of the alert line into the transfer zone and to the action line of the active phase. For normal nulliparous women the augmentation and caesarean section rates left of the alert line were 0.9% and 3.0%, in the transfer zone 4.7% and 8.2%, and at or beyond the action line 25.3% and 64.4%, respectively. The proportions of these interventions in the three time zones for the multiparas were 0.3% and 1.1%, 2.0% and 10.0%, and 16.5% and 66.5%, respectively. Throughout, multiparas had lower caesarean section rates than did nulliparas, but the differences in rates at different parts of the partograph were striking for all parities. The alert and action lines clearly distinguish those labours with an increased likelihood of augmentation and/or operative intervention, and the trial showed that the action line, 4 h parallel to the alert line, should be maintained and that the division between latent and active phase should stay at 3 cm, with the start of the active phase at 3 cm.

An attempt was made in the analysis to distinguish more clearly between women in need of referral once they entered the transfer zone. It was found that entering the referral zone was of significance, regardless of the cervical dilatation. However, if the fetal head was three-fifths or more palpable abdominally when the transfer zone had been reached, caesarean section was a more likely mode of delivery than if the head was two-fifths or less. With the greater likelihood of caesarean section birth when the head is three-fifths or more palpable above the brim in the transfer zone, when the progress of labour moves to the right of the alert line every effort should be made to refer the woman to a unit equipped for operative delivery. The woman's partograph should go with her so that the hospital staff can view her progress in the peripheral unit until transfer. This promotes continuity of care and avoids starting a new partograph in the referral hospital. It is good practice that the staff in the periphery receive encouragement about transfer decisions and are informed of the outcome of the labour by the hospital staff.

CONCLUSIONS ON THE IMPLEMENTATION OF THE PARTOGRAPH

Any labour attendant who can read and perform a vaginal examination should be helped to use a partograph and be given very clear guidelines for management and referral. The strategy advocated is that in any area implementation of the partograph should always commence in the referral hospital. Once the staff there feel comfortable, the partograph should be introduced to peripheral health facilities, with supervision and support from staff at the referral hospital.

It is clear that the introduction of the partograph in this trial has improved hospital practice and its use is universally advocated in all labour wards. The visual recording of the progress of labour strengthens interpretation of labour progress, enhances team work, and improves the care a woman and her unborn child receive during this critical time of labour. With the rise in caesarean section rates (Thiery and Derome, 1986), it is interesting that in this trial prolonged labour, caesarean section rates, and oxytocin augmentation were all reduced without compromising fetal outcome. The reduction of caesarean sections was mainly due to better diagnosis of CPD, supporting the thesis that this is done optimally during a carefully controlled trial of labour with a partograph and a management protocol.

Midwives and physicians who participated in the trial were very pleased with the improved outcomes: increased comfort for women, fewer vaginal examinations, less oxytocin infusions, more time to give care, and the reward of fewer asphyxiated babies, so babies could be bonded and breastfed earlier (Lennox and Kwast, 1995). The partograph should be used for all women who are 'allowed to labour', e.g., those with breech presentation, multiple pregnancy, induction of labour, and medical conditions, as well as women in normal labour. The same labour protocol was used for breech presentation in the multicentre trial, but with the caution that caesarean section may be indicated at the action line. Obstetric staff who are using the partograph for the first time should be reminded that oxytocin augmentation should not be started between alert and action line unless there are special reasons. The interventions are generally guided by the rate of cervical dilatation against the passage of time. Rigid adherence to a protocol should never reduce attention to the general condition of the mother and the fetus. *It is a wise and safe rule not to augment a labour with oxytocin in a health institution without operative facilities, lest disaster strikes with irreversible consequences.*

THE CLINICAL DIAGNOSIS AND MANAGEMENT OF OBSTRUCTED LABOUR

Clinical Diagnosis

Any attendant who does not have a partograph should be taught to recognize lack of progress of labour when there is delay in dilatation (<1 cm/h) and failure of the presenting part to descend. *In the presence of good uterine contractions, cervical arrest of dilatation over 4 h, and increased moulding and caput of the presenting part are usually a sign of impending obstruction.* While this complication should not normally occur in a supervised labour, midwives are presented with women in obstructed labour and need to know how to diagnose the condition.

GENERAL EXAMINATION

The woman is usually dehydrated, anxious, and restless, a condition which is referred to as 'maternal distress'. Genital tract infection is usually present and the woman may have a high fever, tachycardia, and offensive liquor amnii, meconium, or discharge. If signs of shock are present it may be due to severe intrapartum sepsis or a ruptured uterus. A woman with a ruptured uterus may not necessarily have vaginal bleeding if the presenting part is jammed in the pelvis, thus acting as a tampon. The vulva may be oedematous from prolonged pushing. Urine is scanty, concentrated, and in severe cases blood-stained as the bladder becomes congested or if there is already trauma.

ABDOMINAL EXAMINATION

On inspection of the abdomen the bladder may appear to be full, but the soft mass above the symphysis pubis is due to oedema of the bladder. The fundus of the uterus may be felt at the xiphisternum due to excessive thickening and rising of the upper segment. The uterus may still be contracting strongly or, as is usually the case in the primigravida, it may be in a tonic state. The patient feels pain all the time and the lower segment is tender to touch. The level of the presenting part is difficult to feel, but an attempt should be made to define the level of the head in a vertex presentation, because ascertaining the level of the head in relation to the ischial spines on vaginal examination may be misleading due to severe moulding and caput. Sometimes there is evidence of external pressure on the abdomen from attempts to deliver the baby.

There may be severe fetal distress and the maternal pulse rate should always be compared with the fetal heart rate. In this case, with a tachycardic mother, what is interpreted as a fetal heart may well be the maternal souffle. Often the fetal heart will be absent or seriously slow from prolonged intrauterine asphyxia.

VAGINAL EXAMINATION

The vulva may be oedematous and evidence of traditional treatment at home may be detected, such as the insertion of herbs or a 'gishiri' cut. The cervix may be fully dilated in the case of vertex presentation, but it may be oedematous and loosely applied in a neglected transverse lie or breech presentation.

Management of obstructed labour

Obstructed labour is an obstetric emergency and a midwife's skills to provide immediate obstetric first aid are vital. Many countries are recognizing the need to upgrade midwives' and physicians' skills to provide emergency obstetric care, which is part of the seven essential obstetric functions WHO frames in an effort to reduce maternal mortality (WHO, 1991).

IN THE HEALTH CENTRE AND/OR HEALTH POST

If the midwife in the health centre or health post is the first point of contact, every effort should be made to transfer the woman as speedily as possible to a referral hospital, while resuscitative measures are started. *These can save lives and should be undertaken by every midwife practising alone.* It is crucial, therefore, that the midwife recognizes the seriousness of this condition and communicates with the patient and the family in a sympathetic way in order not to apportion blame in such a hazardous situation.

First aid measures include:

1. Starting intravenous infusion to correct dehydration. It is recommended that blood be taken for grouping and cross-matching, if possible, so that the specimen can be taken with the patient to the hospital. Family members should be given an explanation about the necessity for possible blood transfusion, and potential donors should travel with the woman.
2. Broad spectrum antibiotics should be given intramuscularly or intravenously, according to local protocol.
3. Even if the patient's bladder is full, catheterization may be difficult and should be delayed until hospital admission. *A metal catheter should never be used.*
4. Once transport has been arranged, the patient should be accompanied to hospital by the midwife, if possible.

IN HOSPITAL

The same measures as given above should be carried out. In addition, a nasogastric tube should be passed before general anaesthesia. The physician makes the decision as to whether an operation should be carried out to relieve the obstruction. This depends on the condition of the patient, the pelvic capacity, any suspicion of imminent rupture of the uterus, the presentation of the fetus, and whether it is alive or not. The relevant procedures are described by Lawson (1967) and Philpott (1982).

Follow-up care

It is of the utmost importance to support a woman who has experienced obstructed labour, in order to restore her health and self-esteem, and to help her cope with her grief and discomfort. Once recovery is progressing, the past events and plans for the future should be discussed with her and her family. Contraceptive advice and services should be offered if further pregnancies are planned. Care during subsequent pregnancy and delivery needs to be talked about in sufficient detail to convince the woman and her family that care in hospital is required the next time.

CONCLUSIONS

In this chapter the dimensions of prolonged and obstructed labour and the problems which can result in the absence of skilled midwifery and obstetric care have been described. At the threshold of the twenty-first century attempts to reduce prolonged labour and prevent obstructed labour need to be addressed vigorously. This requires a team effort, communication between families and obstetric care givers at all levels of the health service, and referral links for facilities with staff who are trained to deal with the complications and are supported by a reliable drug and supply system. Making motherhood safer does not only consist of safe birth care, but also of improving conditions for the millions of women who labour alone, afar and afraid, who may be deprived of that miraculous culmination of pregnancy – a live and healthy baby.

REFERENCES

Abdullah, S.A., Aboloyoun, E.M., Abdel Aleem, H., Moftah, F.M., and Ismail, S. (1992) Maternal mortality in Assiut. *International Journal of Gynecology and Obstetrics*, **39**: 197–204.

Aitken, I.W. and Walls, B. (1986) Maternal height and cephalopelvic disproportion in Sierra Leone. *Tropical Doctor*, **16**: 132–136.

Alauddin, M. (1986) Maternal mortality in rural Bangladesh. The Tangail District. *Studies in Family Planning*, **17**(1): 13–21.

Alisjahbana, A., Williams, C., Dharmayanti, R., Hermawan, D., Kwast, B.E., and Koblinsky, M. (1995) An integrated village maternity service to improve referral patterns and perinatal mortality in a rural Area in West Java. *International Journal of Obstetrics and Gynaecology*, **48** (Suppl.): S83–S94.

Balde, M.D. and Bastert, G. (1990) Decrease in uterine rupture in Conakry, Guinea, by improvement in transfer management. *International Journal of Gynecology and Obstetrics*, **31**: 21–24.

Basu, S. (1977) Maternity Care in India – An analysis of obstetric deliveries in selected hospitals. In: *India Fertility Research Programme (IFRP)*. Fifth Contributors' Conference, Calcutta. IFRP, New Dehli, India.

Begum, S.F., Nahar, K., Jahan, F.A., and Khan, A.R. (1981) *A comprehensive study of pattern of maternity care services in different hospitals and clinics in Bangladesh*. Presented at the 8th Asian and Oceanic Congress of Obstetrics and Gynecology, October 25–31, 1981.

Bhatia, J.C. (1993) Levels and causes of maternal mortality in Southern India. *Studies in Family Planning*, **24**(5): 310–318.

Bhuiyan, A.B., Ahmed, G., and Rahman, S. (1980) Maternity cases at Rangput Medical College Hospital. In: *Bangladesh Fertility Research Programme (BFRP)*. Fifth Contributors' Conference, Dacca, Bangladesh. BFRP, Dacca, Bangladesh, pp 57–68.

Bird, G.C. (1978) Cervicographic management of labour in primigravidae and multigravidae with vertex presentation. *Tropical Doctor*, **8**: 78–84.

Brennan, M. and Umoh, E. (1993) Training Traditional Birth Attendants. In: *Proceedings of the 23rd Triennial Conference*. International Confederation of Midwives, London.

Center for Population Options (CPO) (1992) *Adolescents and Unsafe Abortions in Developing Countries*. CPO, Washington, DC.

Combs, C.A., Murphy, E.L., and Laros, R.K. (1992) Factors associated with postpartum haemorrhage with vaginal birth. *Obstetrics and Gynaecology*, **77**: 69–76.

Eidelman, A.I., Kamar R., Schimmel M.S., and Baron E. (1988) The grand multipara: is she still a risk? *American Journal of Obstetrics and Gynecology*, **158**: 389–392.

Elbourne, D.R., Prendiville, W.J., and Chalmers, I. (1988) Choice of oxytocic preparation for routine use in the management of the third stage of labour: an overview of the evidence from controlled trials. *British Journal of Obstetrics and Gynaecology*, **95**: 17–30.

Family Health International (1988) *Pregnancy Care Monitoring: Karawa Health Zone, Zaire*. Research Triangle Park, North Carolina.

Friedman, E.A. (1955) Primigravid labour. A graphicostatistical analysis. *Obstetrics and Gynaecology*, **6**(6): 567–589.

Gilbert, L., Porter, W., and Brown, V.A. (1987) Postpartun haemorrhage – a continuing problem. *British Journal of Obstetrics and Gynaecology*, **94**: 67–71.

Iloabachie, G.C. and Agwu, S. (1990) The increasing incidence and declining mortality of ruptured uterus in Enugu. *Journal of Obstetrics and Gynaecology*, **10**: 306–311.

Janowitz, B., Lewis, J., Burton, N., and Lamptey, P. (1984) *Reproductive Health in Africa: Issues and Options*. Family Health International, Research Triangle Park, North Carolina.

Kane, T.T., El Kady, A.A., Saleh, S., Hage, M., Stanback, J., and Potter, L. (1992) Maternal mortality in Giza, Egypt: Magnitude, causes and prevention. *Studies in Family Planning*, **23**(1): 45–57.

Kavoo-Linge and Rogo, K.O. (1992) Factors influencing early perinatal mortality in a rural district hospital. *East African Medical Journal*, **69**(4): 181–187.

Kelly, J. (1992) Audit of health services in Gurage. *Journal of Tropical Pediatrics*, **38**(4): 206–207.

Kelly, J. and Kwast, B.E. (1993) Epidemiologic study of vesicovaginal fistulas in Ethiopia. *International Urogynecology Journal*, **4**: 278–281.

Khan, A.R. (1986) Maternal mortality in rural Bangladesh. The Jamalpur district. *Studies in Family Planning*, **17**(1): 7–12.

Konje, J.C., Obisesan, K.A., and Ladipo, O.A. (1992) Obstructed labor in Ibadan. *International Journal of Gynecology and Obstetrics*, **39**(1): 17–21.

Kumar, R., Sharma, A.K., Barik, S., and Kumar, V. (1989) Maternal mortality inquiry in a rural community of North India. *International Journal of Gynecology and Obstetrics*, **29**(4): 313–319.

Kwast, B.E. (1988) The confidential enquiries. In: Kwast, B.E. (ed.), *Unsafe Motherhood, A Monumental Challenge*. Leiderdorp, The Netherlands, pp 116–136.

Kwast, B.E. (1992) Obstructed labour, its contribution to maternal mortality. *Midwifery*, **8**: 3–7.

Kwast, B.E. (1993) Safe motherhood - the first decade. *Midwifery*, **9**: 105–123.

Lachman, E., Moodley, J., Pitsoe, S.B., and Philpott, R.H. (1985) Rupture of the gravid uterus. *South African Medical Journal*, **67**: 333–338.

Lawson, J.B. (1967) Obstructed labour. In: J.B. Lawson and D.B. Stewart (eds), *Obstetrics and Gynaecology in the Tropics*. Edward Arnold, London, pp 172–218.

Lennox, C.E. and Kwast, B.E. (1995) The partograph in community obstetrics. *Tropical Doctor*, **25**(2): 56–63.

Liljestrand, J., Bergström, S., and Westman, S. (1985) Maternal height and perinatal outcome in Moçambique. *Journal of Tropical Paediatrics*, **31**: 306–310.

Lindpainter, L.S. (1982) *Maternal Mortality in Matlabthana, Bangladesh*. International Centre for Diarrhoeal Diseases Research, Dhaka, Bangladesh.

Liskin, L.S. (1992) Maternal morbidity in developing countries: a review and comments. *International Journal of Obstetrics and Gynaecology*, **37**: 77–87.

Maine, D. (1991) *Safe Motherhood Programs: Options and Issues*. Center for Population and Family Health, Columbia University, New York.

Mola, G. and Aitkin, I. (1984) Maternal mortality in Papua New Guinea, 1976–1983. *Papua New Guinea Medical Journal*, **27**(2): 65–71.

MotherCare (1994) *MotherCare, Lessons Learned 1989–1993.* John Snow, Inc., Arlington, Virginia.

O'Driscoll, K., Stronge, J.M., and Minogue, M. (1973) Active management of labour. *British Medical Journal,* **3**: 135–138.

O'Rourke, K. (1995) An evaluation of a TBA training program: its effect on TBA practices and perinatal mortality. *Bull Pan Am Health Organ* (in press).

Osefo, N.J. (1989) Cesarean and postpartum hysterectomy in Enugu, 1973–1986. *International Journal of Gynaecology and Obstetrics,* **30**(2): 93–97.

Ozumba, B.C. and Uchegbu, H. (1991) Incidence and management of obstructed labour in eastern Nigeria. *Australian and New Zealand Journal of Obstetrics and Gynaecology,* **31**(3): 213–216.

Philpott, R.H. (1982) The recognition of cephalopelvic disproportion. In: Philpott, R.H. (ed.), *Clinics in Obstetrics and Gynaecology.* W.B. Saunders Ltd, London, pp 609–624.

Philpott, R.H. and Castle, W.M. (1972a) Cervicographs in the management of labour in primigravidae. I: The alert line for detecting abnormal labour. *Journal of Obstetris and Gynaecology of the British Commonwealth,* **79**: 592–598.

Philpott, R.H. and Castle, W.M. (1972b) Cervicographs in the management of labour in primigravidae. II: The action line and treatment of abnormal labour. *Journal of Obstetrics and Gynaecology of the British Commonwealth,* **79**: 599–602.

Pillai, G. (1993) *Reducing Deaths from Pregnancy and Childbirth. Asia.* Links Health and Development Report, Washington, D.C.

Poovan, P., Kifle, F., and Kwast, B.E. (1990) A maternity waiting home reduces obstetric catastrophes. *World Health Forum,* **2**: 440–445.

Prendiville, W.J., Elbourne, D.R., and Stirrat G.M. (1988) The Bristol Third Stage Trial: Active versus physiological management of third stage of labour. *British Medical Journal,* **297**: 1295–1300.

Price, T.G. (1984) Preliminary report on maternal deaths in the South Highlands of Tanzania in 1983. *Journal of Obstetrics and Gynaecology of East and Central Africa,* **3**: 103–110.

Public Opinion Polls (1993) *MotherCare Nigeria Maternal Healthcare Project Qualitative Research.* Working Paper: 17B. MotherCare, Arlington, Virginia.

Roosmalen, van J. and Brand, R. (1992) Maternal height and outcome of labor in rural Tanzania. *International Journal of Gynecology and Obstetrics,* **37**: 169–177.

Schieber, B.A. and Szasdi, J.A. (1994) *A Community Surveillance System in Quetzaltenango Health Area, Guatemala.* Internal Publication, INCAP, Guatemala City.

Studd, J. (1973) Partograms and nomograms of cervical dilatation in management of primigravid labour. *British Medical Journal,* **4**: 451–455.

Thiery, M. and Derom, R. (1986) Review of evaluation studies on caesarean section. Part I: Trends in caesarean section and perinatal mortality. In: Kaminsky, M., Breart, G., Buekens, P., Huisies, H.J.M., McIlwaire, G., and Selbmann, M.K. (eds), *Perinatal Care Delivery Systems: Description and Evaluation in European Community Countries.* Oxford University Press, Oxford.

Urrio, T.F. (1991) Maternal deaths at Songea Regional Hospital, Southern Tanzania. *East African Medical Journal,* **68**(2): 81–87.

WHO (1989) *The Prevention and Treatment of Obstetric Fistulae.* WHO/FHE/89.5, WHO, Geneva.

WHO (1991) *Essential Elements of Obstetric Care at First Referral Level.* WHO, Geneva.

WHO (1993a) *The Partograph. A Managerial Tool for the Prevention of Prolonged Labour.* Section I: the principle and strategy. Section II: a user's manual. Section III: facilitator's manual. WHO/FHE/MSM 93.8, 93.9, and 93.10, WHO, Geneva.

WHO (1993b) *Coverage of Maternity Care. A Tabulation of Available Information,* 3rd edn. WHO/FHE/MSM/93.7, WHO, Geneva.

WHO (1994a) World Health Organization partograph in management of labour. *Lancet*, **343**: 1399–1404.

WHO (1994b) *The Application of the WHO Partograph in the Management of Labour.* WHO/FHE/MSM 94.4, WHO, Geneva.

CHAPTER

2

Why is Haemorrhage a Major Cause of Maternal Death? A Case Study of Operational Research in Ghana

Susan Ama Opoku

INTRODUCTION

Databases on maternal mortality in many developing countries are rare and often incomplete and inaccurate, making it difficult to address policy issues. In the mid-1980s there was an urgent need in Africa for community-based research on maternal mortality. Most studies up to that time were descriptive and hospital-based, thereby excluding the large number of maternal deaths that occurred outside hospital. Furthermore, they lacked information on the social, economic, and cultural factors that contributed to maternal ill-health and death, and were not designed to develop, institute, or evaluate preventive measures (Carnegie Corporation New York, 1993). In the past decade a growing number of community-based studies have attempted to provide data on maternal mortality and make recommendations for intervention. One such initiative is the Prevention of Maternal Mortality network.

The Prevention of Maternal Mortality network

After the Safe Motherhood Initiative conference held in Nairobi, Kenya, in February 1987, a team from the Center for Population and Family Health, Columbia University in New York, set up a Maternal Mortality Operations Research project, now known as the Prevention of Maternal Mortality (PMM) network.

The PMM network involves three countries in West Africa: Nigeria, Sierra Leone, and Ghana. A total of 11 teams are employed, each with a focus on one of the five direct causes of maternal deaths, namely, obstructed labour, maternal haemorrhage, sepsis, abortion, and hypertensive diseases of pregnancy.

The overall objectives of the network are:

- To investigate the different causes of maternal death, especially those unrelated to obstetric and medical causes.
- To find sustainable interventions to reduce the misfortune of healthy lives lost.

PMM network research projects are divided into two phases: a planning phase and an implementation or intervention phase. The planning phase, lasting a maximum of 12 months, collates information on the nature of obstetric complications in the research area. This information can be used as a baseline to evaluate future interventions.

Findings from the planning phase are used to develop strategies and make recommendations to improve the survival of pregnant women, particularly in rural communities. This second phase lasts for approximately 3 years, during which continuous monitoring and evaluation are carried out.

A multidisciplinary approach has been adopted by the PMM network, bringing together expertise from four different disciplines: obstetrics and gynaecology, midwifery, community health, and social science. Biostatisticians and other experts are co-opted to the teams when necessary.

In 1988, the University of Ghana Medical School (UGMS) in Accra and the School of Medical Sciences of the University of Science and Technology (SMS-UST) in Kumasi were selected for participation in the PPM network. UGMS chose to examine the problem of maternal mortality due to obstructed labour, while the SMS-UST chose to look at maternal haemorrhage. The rest of this chapter describes operational research carried out to identify the causes of maternal haemorrhage in Kumasi and to propose feasible interventions to reduce maternal mortality as a result of haemorrhage.

THE PMM NETWORK RESEARCH PROJECT IN KUMASI
Background

Ashanti Region is one of 10 administrative regions in Ghana. It has 18 districts, of which Kumasi District is the regional capital.

SMS-UST selected the Ejisu Health District (comprising Ejisu–Juaben and Bosomtwe Atwima Kwanwoma Districts) as the research area because the Juaben Health Centre, which serves as a teaching centre for medical students from SMS-UST and student midwives, is located there. Ejisu District had a projected population of 223,632 in 1988, with a growth rate of 2.6% per annum (Ministry of Health, Ghana, 1988). The district has a poor road network and transportation is limited and private. Telephone services are non-existent and there are only six post offices in a district with over 160 communities.

Ejisu District has one district hospital run by a mission, 21 health centres, and eight primary health stations. The Juaben Health Centre is 30 km from Kumasi, while the mission hospital is about 20 km from Kumasi. Each of these has a resident medical officer.

The hospital and health centre suffer from a shortage of supplies and equipment, essential drugs, and nurses to deal with obstetric emergencies. The majority of emergencies are therefore referred to the Komfo Anokye Teaching Hospital (KATH), Kumasi District, or to Agogo Hospital in a neighbouring district.

Two health centres, Juaben and Kuntenase, were chosen as primary referral levels in the project. The secondary referral point was the mission hospital and the tertiary referral point was KATH.

In 1988, maternal mortality in Ghana was estimated to be 5–10 per 1000 live births, and haemorrhage associated with pregnancy and labour was the leading cause of maternal death. Hospital-based data from Kumasi revealed that postpartum haemorrhage accounted for 27.4% of maternal deaths (Ministry of Health, Ghana, 1989). Maternal mortality in Ejisu District was estimated to be about 10–15/1000 live births (Ministry of Health, Ghana, 1988). There was no information at the district level on the incidence of haemorrhage, but it was assumed that the picture would be similar to that of the region as a whole. Maternal haemorrhage was chosen as the focus of PMM research in Kumasi because of the high contribution that it made to overall maternal mortality in the region.

A *maternal death* is defined, according to the World Health Organization (WHO) and the International Federation of Gynaecology and Obstetrics, as the death of a woman while pregnant or within 42 days of termination of pregnancy, irrespective of the duration and the site of the pregnancy, from any cause related to or aggravated by the pregnancy or its management, but not from accidental or incidental causes.

A case was classified as *maternal haemorrhage* if a woman experienced abnormal bleeding of any kind during pregnancy, delivery, or puerperium.

Four different methods of collecting data were used: focus group discussions, a community health survey, an institutional survey, and a time and motion study. Field work took place between December 1989 and June 1990.

Focus group discussions

Focus group discussions were carried out in December 1989. The objective of the focus group discussions was to provide an overall picture of community knowledge, attitudes, beliefs, and practices on:

- Causes of maternal haemorrhage.
- Management of maternal haemorrhage.
- Effectiveness of management.
- Obstacles to obtaining and receiving care.
- Feasible strategies for helping to reduce preventable maternal deaths.

METHODOLOGY

Four teams were trained in focus group discussion techniques. In order to ensure consistency, a focus group guide was developed, which was translated into the local language, 'Twi'. All discussions were conducted in 'Twi' and were recorded on tape with the consent of participants. Sessions lasted between 90 and 20 minutes. A total of 20 focus group discussions were conducted, with participants selected according to age, occupation, and status in the community (*Figure 2.1*).

Social group	Age range	No. of sessions	Participants per session
Teenage mothers	14–19	2	8
Young mothers	20–25	3	10
Female adults	35+	4	8
ANC attendants	16–30	1	11
TBAs/ Queenmothers	55–80	5	6
Male (youth)	20–28	1	10
Male teachers	30–45	2	12
Fathers living with family	30+	2	8

ANC = Antenatal clinic.
TBA = Traditional birth attendant.

Figure 2.1 Characteristics of focus group sessions by social group, age range, and number of participants.

RESULTS

Recognition of complications

Almost all participants could give an example of a complication of pregnancy. Typically, antepartum haemorrhage and postpartum haemorrhage, obstructed labour, and retained placenta were mentioned. Postpartum haemorrhage was described as a life-threatening condition which resulted in death. Participants said that after birth a woman lost about '2 mineral bottles of blood' (300 ml/bottle), but that when the blood loss increased and began to pour 'like a pipe' they knew that something was wrong. However, they did not consider antepartum haemorrhage as serious, because it did not result in immediate death.

Causes of maternal haemorrhage

As *Figure 2.2* shows, 19 possible causes of maternal haemorrhage were mentioned, of which punishment for infidelity, multiparity, a fall during pregnancy, and retained placenta were the four most frequently mentioned.

Traditional management of maternal haemorrhage

It was widely agreed that in cases of maternal haemorrhage advice was first sought from traditional healers and fetish priests. Healers and priests are believed to have magical powers drawn from a deity and are able to make a person disclose hidden secrets. Only after a confession has been extracted is traditional management carried out or alternative care sought. Fear of dying may force some women to confess to things that they have not done, in order to get help.

Remedies

Figure 2.3 summarizes some common local preparations and other methods of management. The methods noted are commonly used by TBAs, Queenmothers, and adult females, who normally attend to deliveries.

Causes of maternal haemorrhage	Young mothers	Female adults	ANC attendants	Male teachers	TBAs/Queen-mother	Male youth	Fathers	Teen mothers
Multiparity			+	+		+	+	
Weak uterus				+			+	
Increased work-load						+		
Fall during pregnancy	+		+	+	+	+		+
Refusing salt-free diet								
Diseases, e.g. jaundice		+						
Punishment for infidelity	+	+	+	+	+		+	+
Hypertension				+				
High protein diet		+			+			+
Anaemia				+				
Retained placenta		+	+		+		+	
Fever/malaria		+	+		+			
Too much sex		+			+			
Severe dysmenorrhoea		+						
Narrow hips				+				
Wide gap between pregnancies	+							
Refusal to attend ANC	+					+		
Ectopic pregnancy								+
Malposition of fetus								+

+ = Cause mentioned by group.

Figure 2.2 Community focus group research on causes of maternal haemorrhage.

Traditional management of maternal haemorrhage	Young mothers	Female adults	ANC attendants	Male teachers	TBAs/Queen-mother	Male youth	Fathers	Teen mothers
Oral preparations								
Starch solutions		+						
Mixture of soot and salt		+			+		+	
Herbal drink					+			
Powdered okra seeds					+			
Pawpaw roots, salt and water		+						
Plantain products								
Fresh roasted plantain leaves as towel pad	+		+		+			+
Two fingers of ripe plantain (eaten)	+	+			+		+	+
Roasted green plantain (eaten)		+			+		+	+
Others								
Patient taken to fetish priest		+			+			
Patient blows air into bottle					+			

+ = Cause mentioned by group.

Figure 2.3 Community focus group research on practices in the management of maternal haemorrhage.

Effectiveness of traditional management

Participants reported that the traditional methods they employed were useful, but if bleeding continued, alternative measures were taken, usually to seek modern medical care.

Little is known about whether traditional methods employed are harmful, innocuous, or potentially beneficial, as none has been tested scientifically. However, many of these practices are time consuming and may cause delay in seeking modern medical care.

FACTORS DELAYING SEEKING MODERN MEDICAL CARE

Transportation

Participants complained of lack of regular transport to convey patients to health facilities. In some villages there were no vehicles at all, or there was only one vehicle which left at dawn and returned at nightfall, while others had access to transport once a week, usually on a market day. A woman with a postpartum haemorrhage or other obstetric complication would either be carried in a hammock to the nearest health facility or be left to die.

Roads in Ejisu District are poor and during the rainy season may become flooded and muddy, preventing the movement of vehicles. In very remote villages, footpaths are the only link with roads. Participants reported that drivers were unwilling to soil their vehicles with blood and most refused to carry a bleeding woman. Concern was voiced that even when a driver agreed to take a woman to a health facility, the uneven road caused great pain and could potentially worsen her condition. Nearly all participants mentioned the cost of transport and that in an emergency some drivers increased the cost of transportation.

The community and health workers complained that health centres did not have ambulances to convey patients referred to hospital. Families incurred an additional cost in time and money if they decided to go to the hospital. Some patients never reached the hospital because they died en route. Alternatively, families decided to send the patient back to her village rather than incur additional cost and disappointment.

Health service factors

Participants reported that the staff at out-patient departments could be unhelpful. Some staff were described as 'rude', 'impatient', or 'with no sense of urgency'. After registration in the out-patient department, some women had to wait in a queue in spite of having reported the postpartum haemorrhage; also, limited theatre space meant waiting for operations.

Hospital fees, purchase of drugs and blood, and upkeep of relatives accompanying the patient to a health facility were mentioned as financial barriers to seeking prompt medical care.

Drugs, equipment, and supplies were reported to be in short supply or not available and relatives were required to go outside the hospital to buy medical items. Often they did not have money for such purchases, leading to further delay in care.

It was claimed that a long and tedious process was involved in getting blood from the blood bank services at the hospital. There was almost always a shortage of blood in the blood bank and blood was sold privately at often unaffordable prices.

CONCLUSIONS

The experiences outlined above are not unique to the Ghanaian situation. Two Nigerian studies have also identified service shortcomings, such as staff rudeness, long waiting times, shortage of drugs and supplies, distance, transport costs, and the costs of being away from home, as reasons for non-utilization of health services (Stock, 1983; Bamisaiye *et al.*, 1986).

Institutional factors may actually contribute to worsening an already bad situation. Studies by Hickey and Kasonde (1977) in Lusaka, Zambia, on maternal mortality in health facilities indicate that the bulk of institutional maternal mortality is avoidable.

The focus group discussions suggest that the death of a woman from haemorrhage in pregnancy or childbirth is not the result only of obstetric complication, but is multifactorial.

Community survey on maternal health, morbidity, and mortality

A community-based survey on maternal health, illness, and death was carried out in January and February of 1990. The survey further investigated the management of obstetric emergencies, traditional practices, and factors associated with maternal deaths in the community.

METHODOLOGY

Of 160 communities, 80 were selected (using a cluster sampling method) to take part in the survey. The survey was carried out by Ministry of Health staff under the supervision of the research team. Interviewers were trained in face-to-face interviewing techniques using questionnaires and the interviews were conducted in 'Twi'. Data on obstetric emergencies, including maternal mortality due to haemorrhage, were gathered.

On arrival at each community, interviewers proceeded to the central part of the village and spun a pointed object. They then entered the first house in the direction of the pointer and asked to interview all women present who were in the fertile age-group. They then selected the next house whose door was nearest to them and continued in this fashion until they obtained the requisite number of interviews for the given community.

Where a woman who had died in pregnancy, delivery, or the puerperium was identified, the next-of-kin, usually the sister or uncle, was visited to obtain more details about her death.

RESULTS

Maternal death

For the period January 1985 to December 1989, 50 maternal deaths were identified. The results presented here are based on the 44 maternal deaths for which relevant data were obtained.

Of the women who died, 59% (26) were aged between 20 and 34 years, while 41% (18) were in the high-risk age groups (less than 20 years or 35 years and above); 81.8% (36) were married and 45.4% (20) had an average of three living children at the time of death; 63.8% (28) had at least primary education. Their major occupations were farmers, housewives, and seamstresses.

Year	Number of deaths	Estimated births
1985	9	4617
1986	10	4737
1987	7	4860
1988	6	4986
1989	12	5116
Total	**44**	**24,316**

Figure 2.4 Number of maternal deaths identified during the community survey, and estimated births, 1985–1989.

Estimated maternal mortality

The number of deaths for each year covered by the survey are shown in *Figure 2.4*. The average estimated maternal mortality rate based on a district crude birth rate of 40/1000 population (Ghana Statistical Services, 1989) was 181/100,000 total births per year.

Presumptive causes of maternal death

The main causes of maternal mortality reported were postpartum haemorrhage (20), jaundice in pregnancy (10), obstructed labour (3), eclampsia (3), and fever presumed to be malaria (5). The others were ectopic pregnancy, abortions, and antepartum haemorrhage.

Factors associated with maternal death

- *Antenatal care.* Of the women who died, 34% (15) did not receive antenatal care during their most recent pregnancy, 32% (14) made between five and nine antenatal visits, and 34% (15) were reported to have made more than 10 antenatal visits.
- *Place of maternal death.* About 68% (30) of the women died after reaching a health facility, 27% (12) died at home while being attended to by family members, and 4.5% (2) died under the care of untrained local traditional birth attendants. A little over two-thirds of the women died during delivery or in the first 6 h after the baby was born.

Maternal health, morbidity, and service use

1200 women aged between 15 and 49 were interviewed in the 80 communities. Of the women interviewed, about 60% had at least primary education and 50% had married at under 20 years.

About 70% of the women reported that they attended antenatal clinics at least four times in their most recent pregnancy. The target for maternal health in Ghana is at least four antenatal visits in any one pregnancy (Ministry of Health, 1992). Asked why they attended the clinic, some of the following reasons were given:

- To determine position of baby.
- To detect abnormalities early enough for intervention to be made.

- To prevent complications.
- To prevent contracting a disease.
- To get advice on diet.

Family planning
The majority of women (85%) knew about at least one modern family planning method, yet only 5.5% were using one at the time of interview.

Maternity waiting homes
A maternity waiting home is a place near to the hospital provided for women who fall within the identified 'high risk' group when they are close to their dates of confinement. A midwife visits the home at regular intervals to attend to women who stay there.

About 90% of the women interviewed said that they would be willing to stay in a maternity waiting home if advised to do so. Most women said that they would be prepared to stay a month or two. It was impossible to ascertain whether families and family responsibilities would create obstacles to this.

Local treatment for bleeding in pregnancy
Of the respondents, 20% knew about local herbal preparations used as first aid during the management of haemorrhage. They reported that should these fail they would seek treatment at a health facility.

Factors affecting referral of patients to secondary and tertiary referral levels by health-centre staff in the district
Geographical location, both in terms of physical proximity to referral points and linkage with a main road, was a factor in determining referral. Lack of vehicles to convey patients from the health centres to the referral centres and inadequate follow-up by staff were also mentioned as constraining factors.

CONCLUSIONS
The important contribution of haemorrhage, especially postpartum haemorrhage, to high maternal mortality found in the present survey is corroborated by many other community surveys on maternal mortality in developing countries (Greenwood et al., 1987; Walker et al., 1986).

Jaundice in pregnancy, found to be the second major cause of death, may have been due to the use of hepatotoxic herbal enemata, which is a common practice in this rural district. No information on these herbal preparations was available. Other possible causes are malaria, certain blood diseases, and hepatitis. Reports from Accra, Ghana, reveal that women of low socioeconomic status are particularly susceptible to viral hepatitis (Ampofo, 1969).

The findings suggest that antenatal care alone was insufficient to prevent deaths. The 1991 *Annual Maternal and Child Health/Family Planning* report showed that most rural women in Ghana attend antenatal clinic, but deliver at home. A recent survey on maternal mortality in northern Ghana revealed that 70% of all women attended an antenatal clinic at least once during their pregnancy, but that antenatal attendance alone did not improve a woman's chances of survival (Dollimore *et al.*, 1993). A review of the effectiveness of antenatal care in maternal health has been conducted by the Maternal Health and Safe Motherhood Programme of the WHO (Rooney, 1992). It suggests that antenatal care can be effective for conditions for which risk factors are clearly identifiable during pregnancy (e.g., obstructed labour, eclampsia, anaemia, and infections), but, as Thaddeus and Maine (1990) point out, antenatal care alone in a rural setting does very little to prevent or control postpartum haemorrhage.

The physical, socio-cultural, and economic barriers to seeking professional health care may delay the decision to use health services until very late, which may explain in part the high number of deaths in health service facilities. A study by Harrison (1985) in northern Nigeria showed that the non-use of services is associated with higher rates of maternal and perinatal death.

In 1988, fees for hospital delivery were increased throughout the country and pregnant women had to pay for all drugs used during their management. The doubling of the number of deaths in 1989 may have been due to resultant non-utilization of health institutions.

The community survey showed that while women recognized the importance and function of antenatal services, few used modern family planning methods. The reason may be explained partly by the strong pro-birth culture of most rural communities in Ghana. However, it may also be due to an 'unmet need' for family planning services.

Limitations

As the study did not cover all communities in the district, the number of maternal deaths identified may not be representative. It proved impossible to verify data on women reported to have died in a health facility, as it is common practice for patients to give an address of a relative or friend in the town where the facility is located rather than their home address. In addition, most people in this rural district use two names, one for home and another for official records. This makes follow-up difficult! Poor documentation of patients' histories and poor record-keeping in the health institutions compound the problem.

Institutional review

A review of hospital records from the maternity block at KATH was undertaken to determine:

- The number and types of cases of maternal haemorrhage.
- The mortality due to maternal haemorrhage.
- The institutional factors related to and influencing mortality due to maternal haemorrhage.
- The use of findings to reduce mortality due to maternal haemorrhage.

METHODOLOGY

Six years, 1981, 1983, 1985, 1987, 1988, and 1989, were chosen for examination because anecdotal evidence suggested that changes were introduced in these years which affected dramatically the lives of the majority of the people in Ghana. In 1981 there was a change in government rule. In 1983 the country was ravaged by bush fires and famine. In 1985 user charges at Ministry of Health facilities were introduced, with the exception of maternity care. Although 1987 was a relatively uneventful year, in 1988 mothers were asked to pay for delivery and all drugs that were prescribed. In 1989 the Ministry of Health proposed a cash and carry system of drug procurement.

In-patient case notes, labour ward delivery notes, and theatre records of all cases of maternal haemorrhage admitted at the maternity block were examined. Definitions were based on the International Classification of Diseases, ninth and tenth editions. The details of each case were summarized on disease classification index cards and filed for each given year (for further details see Martey *et al.*, 1993).

Cases of maternal haemorrhage that were compiled included all admitted cases of ruptured ectopic pregnancy, threatened and incomplete abortion, and antepartum and postpartum haemorrhage.

RESULTS

As *Figure 2.5* shows, maternal haemorrhage as a percentage of maternity admissions was, on average, 22.2%. Taken as a percentage of deliveries this was, on average, 31.1%, but varied from 27.6% in 1981 to 32.7% in 1989 with a peak of 36.3% in 1983.

Haemorrhage accounted for 27.2% of the total 668 maternal deaths with little yearly variation, except in 1987 when it accounted for 22.4% of deaths. The case fatality rate of maternal haemorrhage decreased from 1.34% in 1981 to 0.7% in 1989.

CONCLUSIONS

A high proportion of maternal deaths attributable to haemorrhage occurred at KATH. Similar results have been reported from Tanzania (Armon, 1979).

	1981	1983	1985	1987	1988	1989
Admissions	12,674	12,379	14,660	14,700	13,187	14,277
Deliveries	9293	8165	10,106	10,711	9447	10,893
Total obstetric complications	6323	6809	6918	6967	5862	7718
Obstetric complications as percentage of deliveries	68	83.4	68.5	65.0	62.1	70.0
Maternal haemorrhage	2561	2965	3356	2911	2881	3564
Maternal haemorrhage as percentage of admission	20.2	23.9	22.9	19.8	21.8	24.9
Maternal haemorrhage as percentage of deliveries	27.6	36.3	33.2	27.2	30.5	32.7
Maternal haemorrhage as percentage of obstetric complications	40.5	43.5	48.5	41.8	49.1	46.2
Maternal deaths	120	123	113	116	105	91
Deaths due to haemorrhage	34	36	33	26	28	25
Percentage of maternal deaths due to haemorrhage	28.3	29.3	29.2	22.4	26.7	27.4
Case fatality rate of maternal haemorrhage (%)	1.34	1.21	0.98	0.89	0.97	0.7

Figure 2.5 Obstetric complications, including those at the maternity block, at KATH for selected years.

The decline in case fatality between 1981 and 1989 may be attributed to a number of factors, including improvements in drug and medical supplies and the establishment of a postgraduate residency programme in obstetrics in 1985 at KATH.

Note that the total number of admissions, deliveries, and obstetric complications at the hospital decreased in 1988 compared to previous years. Maternal haemorrhage as percentage of admissions, deaths due to haemorrhage, and percentage of maternal deaths due to haemorrhage also increased. This may have been due to the introduction of delivery fees, which led women to delay going to hospital until too late.

Time-and-motion study

A time-and-motion study was undertaken in the maternity block at KATH to identify points in the admission process where delays occurred.

METHODOLOGY

The study was based on 153 cases of maternal haemorrhage seen between January 1990 and March 1990. All cases of maternal haemorrhage were followed through from the out-patients' registration to the operating theatre. The time spent at each point and between each point was recorded.

For the purposes of this study, a case was classified as maternal haemorrhage if any of the following diagnoses were listed on the medical card: ruptured ectopic pregnancy, antepartum haemorrhage, postpartum haemorrhage, threatened abortion, and incomplete abortion.

Four points of contact in the hospital were identified as areas where delays might occur: out-patient records department, out-patient consulting room, the maternity ward, and the operating theatre. Four data collection forms for the different points of contact were designed and pre-tested.

Patients were assigned a questionnaire code and at each of the four points a patient's time of arrival, time of departure, and time taken to perform an action were recorded. The forms were completed by specially trained personnel from the Biostatistics Unit of the hospital. The data were compiled and analysed by the research team.

RESULTS

Figure 2.6 shows the average length of time spent at each of the different points. On average, patients spent 5 minutes waiting to be registered at out-patients, 4 minutes waiting to be seen in the consulting room, 10 minutes in the consulting room, and 15 minutes going from the consulting room to the ward. Time spent in the ward varied according to the diagnosis.

CONCLUSIONS

No major cause of delay in the hospital was evident, although some delay was caused by lack of equipment and medical supplies. This may have been due to the presence of the recorders, who stimulated the hospital staff to act more energetically than usual.

The longest delay, ranging from 3 h to whole days, occurred between the onset of symptoms and arrival at the hospital. In the case of illegally induced abortion, one reason for the delay may have been fear of recrimination by the hospital staff.

Point of contact	Average waiting time				
	Ruptured ectopic	Postpartum haemorrhage	Antepartum haemorrhage	Threatened abortion	Complete abortion
OPD (records)	5 m	5 m	7 m	3 m	7 m
Interval between OPD and consulting room	3 m	3 m	4 m	9 m	4 m
Consulting room	13 m	15 m	11 m	6 m	8 m
Interval between consulting room and wards	18 m	28 m	15 m	9 m	8 m
Wards	10 m	1 h 2 m	1 h 8 m	3 h 39 m	4 h 9 m
Arrival at operating theatre (delay time)	49 m	1 h 5 m	1 h 45 m	4 h 6 m	4 h 36 m
Interval between leaving home and arrival at hospital	1 h 12 m	7 h 9 m	14 h 4 m	31 h 10 m	25 h 38 m

OPD = Outpatient Department..

Figure 2.6 Average waiting times by diagnosis.

INTERVENTIONS AND IMPLEMENTATION

The following recommendations for intervention to avoid delay in seeking care and strengthening institutional capacity were proposed.

Community level
- Initiate intensive community health education on the dangers of bleeding in pregnancy and the need to seek appropriate care promptly.
- Educate communities about maternal health care and obstetric emergencies.
- Encourage sharing of transport within and between villages and promote co-operation between village health committees and the local road transport unions to provide transport to women with obstetric emergencies.
- Encourage and establish voluntary blood donor associations in all communities.
- Encourage communities to set up health funds for obstetric emergencies based on a system of prepayments.
- Train and supervise TBAs in aseptic delivery technique and in basic procedures, such as nipple stimulation and uterine massage for women with haemorrhage.
- Encourage communities close to the mission hospital to construct a maternity waiting home.

District and health centre level
- Refurbish theatre at Juaben Health Centre, purchase an operating kit (laparotomy set), and advocate the posting of a resident doctor to manage obstetric emergencies.
- Set up a blood bank at Juaben health centre and establish a 24 h blood service link with KATH.
- Provide and replenish essential drug stocks for obstetric emergencies at all district health centres.
- Train all district midwives (from private and government health institutions) in life-saving skills for obstetric emergencies.
- Train district health staff in interpersonal skills.

- Supervise and assist all trained district TBAs.
- Introduce an 'at risk' register at all district health centres.
- Introduce referral and feedback forms at all district health institutions.

KATH management board
- Provide all wards in the maternity block with resuscitation packs for use in emergencies.
- Introduce a confidential enquiry protocol for all maternal deaths at KATH, Kumasi.

The research team
- Establish a system of maternity-care monitoring at KATH and the mission hospital.
- Provide and maintain essential drug and medical supplies for obstetric emergencies to the district maternity blocks and KATH under the supervision of the research team midwife.

Monitoring and evaluation
Monitoring and evaluation plans were developed to ensure that there were regular assessment of the interventions and to provide adequate and timely information for management decisions.

LESSONS LEARNED
At the time of writing, the PMM project in Kumasi was in its final year of implementation. A number of issues relating to the management and implementation of the project are discussed below.

The use of a multidisciplinary research team
Inputs from the community physician and social scientist proved very useful and educative to team members, especially to the obstetrician and the midwife who had little experience of working in a community or outside the hospital environment. It is recommended that such a multidisciplinary approach be adopted for any similar projects.

Field trips to the remote parts of the district
Trips to remote villages were exhausting, but illustrated the obstacles that villagers have to overcome in emergencies. As the project progressed, field trips became an exciting and valuable experience for all members.

Setbacks
Problems in obtaining funds for the intervention phase of the project caused delays, so loss of interest was a potential problem.

Co-ordination of the research through the university rather than the Ministry of Health had advantages and disadvantages. An advantage was that, as an academic institution, the university was more receptive to undertaking research. A disadvantage, however, was that 80% of team members were Ministry of Health staff and, therefore, obtaining funds from the university to carry out interventions often proved difficult and contributed to delays and frustration. Furthermore, the project was implemented by staff of the Ministry of Health, but the Ministry itself had no major responsibility for the whole project.

It is suggested that future projects of this nature should have resources directed through the Ministry of Health, which should be the implementing organization.

REFERENCES

Ampofo, D.A. (1969) Causes of maternal death and comments: maternity hospital, Accra 1963–1967. *West African Medical Journal*, **18**(3): 75–81.

Armon, P.J. (1979) Maternal deaths in the Kilimanjaro region of Tanzania. *Transactions of the Royal Society of Tropical Medicine and Hygiene*, **73**: 284–288.

Bamisaiye, A., Ransome-Kuti, O., and Famurewa, A.A. (1986) Waiting time and its impact on service acceptability and coverage at an MCH clinic in Lagos, Nigeria. *Journal of Tropical Paediatrics*, **32**(4): 158–161.

Carnegie Corporation New York (1993) Making pregnancy and childbearing safer for women in West Africa. *Carnegie Quarterly*, **38**(1).

Dollimore, N., Odoi-Agyarko, H., and Owusu-Agyei, O. (1993) *A Community Based Study of Risk Factors in Maternal Mortality in the Kassena–Nankana District of Northern Ghana*. Report for the Safe Motherhood Initiative of WHO, Geneva, Contract Number HQ/91/903839.

Ghana Statistical Services (1989) *Ghana Demographic and Health Survey 1988*. IRD/Macro-System, Columbia, Maryland, pp 31–33.

Greenwood, A.M., Greenwood, B.M., Bradley, A.K., Williams, K., Shenton, F.C., Tulloch, S., Byass, P., and Oldfield, F.S.J. (1987) A prospective survey of the outcome of pregnancy in rural area of the Gambia. *Bulletin WHO*, **65**: 635–643.

Harrison, K.A. (1985) Childbearing, health and social priorities: a survey of 22,774 consecutive hospital births in Zaria, Northern Nigeria. *British Journal of Obstetrics and Gynaecology*, **92** (Suppl. 5): 1–119.

Hickey, M.U. and Kasonde, J.M. (1977) Maternal mortality at University Teaching Hospital, Lusaka. *Medical Journal of Zambia*, **11**: 74–78.

Martey, J.O., Djan, J.O., Twum, S., Browne, E.N.L., and Opuku, S.A. (1993) Maternal mortality due to haemorrhage in Ghana. *International Journal of Gynaecology and Obstetrics*, **42**: 237–241.

Ministry of Health, Ghana (1988) *District Health Profile, Ejisu District*. District Health Management Team, Ejisu (mimeograph).

Ministry of Health, Ghana (1989) *Annual Report, Ashanti Region*. Unpublished.

Ministry of Health, Ghana (1992) *Maternal and Child Health/Family Planning Annual National Report, 1991, Accra*. Unpublished.

Rooney, C. (1992) *Antenatal Care and Maternal Health: How Effective Is It?* WHO, Geneva (WHO/MSM/92.4).

Stock, R. (1983) Distance and utilisation of health facilities in rural Nigeria. *Social Science and Medicine*, **17**(19): 363–370.

Thaddeus, S. and Maine, D. (1990) *Too Far To Walk. Maternal Mortality in Context. (Findings from A Multidisciplinary Literature Review)*. Prevention of Maternal Mortality Program, Center for Population and Family Health, Columbia University, New York.

Walker, G.J.A., Ashley, D.E.C., McCaw, A., and Bernard, G.W. (1986) Estimating maternal mortality in Jamaica. *Lancet*, **i**: 486–488.

CHAPTER

3

The Determinants of Maternity Service Utilization in Peri-Urban Communities: A Case Study From Zambia

Esnarst Shakulipa Namakando

INTRODUCTION

Of the world's annual half million maternal deaths, 30% occur in Africa, where as many as eight of every 1000 live births result in maternal death (WHO, 1986), the majority of which are avoidable. The causes of death are complex and usually involve medical, health service, social, and economic factors (WHO, 1986; Kwast, 1989). Lack of both access to and acceptability of maternity services are important contributors to risk. Services may not be available, women may not use them because of ignorance, cost, distance, or time considerations, or because of family and societal pressure. Kwast (1988) suggests that often it is the groups that have the highest mortality (the unmarried primigravidae, the multigravidae, and those from lower socioeconomic groups) who are least likely to use health service facilities. In developing countries, the vast majority of deaths in childbirth occur among emergency admissions of women who had no previous care.

Although the role of antenatal care has been challenged recently by various authors (Tew, 1990; Rooney, 1992), it is likely that it plays a significant role in detecting and providing timely intervention to some of the 'at risk' mothers and to those who are in the early stages of complications. Evidence from Africa suggests that the non-use of antenatal services is associated with a higher risk of maternal mortality. A study of 3414 Zairian women who delivered at a rural hospital between 1981 and 1983 showed that the risk of death was increased 15-fold in women who had not received antenatal care compared with those who had (Mahler, 1987). Two maternal mortality studies carried out at Lusaka's University Teaching Hospital in 1977 and 1986 showed similar associations between maternal death and lack of antenatal care. The cause of death in 50% of the women was hypertensive diseases (Hickey and Kasonde, 1977; Mhango, 1986).

DETERMINANTS OF HEALTH SERVICE UTILIZATION

Several models have been developed over the past two decades to describe the factors that influence health service utilization (Andersen and Newman, 1973; Kohn and White, 1976; Poole and Carlton, 1986; Thaddeus and Maine, 1990). All these models include factors related to the health delivery system ('service factors') and factors related to the potential client ('user factors'). A wide range of societal, economic, and cultural factors are known to influence the latter (Benyoussef and Wessen, 1974).

Service factors

Three distinct 'service factors' are often cited. These are distance, cost, and quality of care.

DISTANCE

The geographical proximity of services to people's homes is one of the most important factors to influence utilization of health services. Long distance and absence of transportation to reach a health facility can be real barriers, even in developed countries. Buekens (1990) cites two North American studies in which not having a car was perceived as a major obstacle to accessing care. In Glasgow, Scotland, Reid and McIlwaine (1980) found that the majority of women would prefer to have a peripheral clinic closer to their homes.

Studies carried out in the developing world indicate that out-patient attendance decreases exponentially with distance (Jolly and King, 1966). In a rural area of Kenya, Voorhoeve (1982) found a decrease in antenatal care attendance from 93% at 8 km to 69% at 24 km from the hospital. In Cebu, the Philippines, rural women made more antenatal visits when clinics were within walking distance (Wong, 1987). Similar findings have been reported from Nigeria (Orubuloye and Caldwell, 1975; Egunjobi, 1983; Stock, 1983; Freeman, 1983) and from Iraq (Habib and Vaughan, 1986).

There is, however, some evidence which suggests that distance is not the only significant factor that determines the clients' use of health services. In Guatemala, Annis (1981) found that some health facilities which had been strategically placed around markets in an effort to attract clients were not used, probably due to the clients' dissatisfaction with the services themselves. In Nigeria, Stock (1983) found that people were prepared to travel long distances in search of what they perceived to be 'quality care'. In Kenya, although the upgrading of the main truck road through Kenya's Meru district significantly reduced travel distance and time, admission rates to the mission hospital did not show a significant improvement (Airey, 1989).

COST

The cost of a service can either be 'direct' (payment for transport, drugs, and user fees), or 'indirect' or 'private' (competing demands on time) (Graham and Campbell, 1990). In developing countries, indirect costs can have an enormous impact because women may have many children to care for and are responsible for all the household work. Observation of such women shows that they have less time to take care of their own health (Pinot and Faundes, 1989). Competing demands on women's time tend to have more serious implications for the uptake of preventive than of curative care, since the former is often perceived as non-essential (Population Reports, 1988). In a village in West Bengal, India, 42% of pregnant women who were interviewed did not use antenatal services, mainly because it took too much time (Ray, 1984). Similar findings were noted by Dor and Gaag (1988) in the Ivory Coast.

In Mexico, lack of money to pay for fees was found to be a critical consideration behind the non-use of physicians in 58% of illness episodes (Young, 1981). In the United States, Frank (1990) found that a significantly lower percentage of uninsured patients were admitted to 'for-profit' hospitals than to secular or church-affiliated, non-profit hospitals and public hospitals.

During the past decade, the issue of user fees has become particularly important in developing countries, where they have been introduced as a form of cost recovery in government services, previously offered free. Although user fees may generate a small amount of revenue for a government, it can deter the utilization of services.

QUALITY OF CARE

Cost, however, like distance, may not always be a major deterrent in seeking care. Two Nigerian studies, by Egunjobi (1983) and Nnadi and Kabat (1984), and one Ethiopian study, by Kloos (1987), showed that people preferred to pay for medical services in the belief that they would receive better care. Thaddeus and Maine (1990) point out that where potential patients have access to more than one facility, their judgement on quality of care often takes precedence over their concerns about cost.

Satisfaction with services received can affect future service utilization. In the developing world, government health facilities often fare worse in terms of client satisfaction than do mission facilities. This could be because mission health facilities are better equipped and staffed, and are therefore able to offer services which better meet the clients' requirements.

The issue of waiting time is also vital. Long waiting lists and long waiting times can impede early antenatal care. Even in developed countries, such as Britain, bureaucratic delay by hospitals in giving appointments can delay early antenatal attendance (Simpson and Walker, 1980).

User factors

A client's perception of the need for care has a significant influence on utilization of health services (Benyoussef and Wessen, 1974). Socio-demographic variables, such as economic status, educational level, parity, and marital status, have all been identified as affecting the utilization of health services. The availability of others to help with household chores, to look after children, or to accompany patients to the facility affect the decision to seek care. A close relationship between social network and utilization has been noted in Nigeria (Stock, 1983) and Iraq (Habib and Vaughan, 1986).

ECONOMIC STATUS

Studies have shown that a high proportion of poor women consistently receive inadequate or no antenatal care. A study by Kwast (1989) in Addis Ababa showed that the use of antenatal care services and of health care facilities for delivery increased significantly with increased economic status. Studies in Iraq (Habib and Vaughan, 1986) and Nigeria (Stock, 1983) reported similar findings.

MATERNAL EDUCATION

Available evidence suggests that a formal education is associated with higher utilization of formal health services, particularly the preventive services. Education provides not only an increased understanding of health needs and of methods of modern medicine, but also allows an individual to develop a more cosmopolitan view of the world. In a New York population, utilization varied according to the degree to which populations demonstrated 'cosmopolitan' as opposed to 'parochial' attitudes (Benyoussef and Wessen, 1974).

This tendency is likely to be even more evident in developing countries, where education, even of a primary level, is a major force in breaking down traditional world views and folk practices. An important function of education is to help individuals cope with their needs by making intelligent use of the available social and health services. Brazilian data show that the proportion of women attending antenatal care clinics was especially low in the less-educated group. This may reflect "ignorance of the advantages of preventive care" (Pinot and Faundes, 1989). In Jordan, Abbas and Walker (1986) found that 76% of women with no formal education were non-users, compared to 30% of those with secondary education.

WOMEN'S STATUS

One important aspect of women's status is their ability to take decisions in relation to their health. In developing countries, many women do not have the power to decide about their health due to cultural constraints. This is well-illustrated in a Senegalese study, in which only 2% of the women interviewed said they would take the decision to seek health care. For 52% of the women, the decision would be made by the husband, while for 44% another family member made the decision (Dia, 1990). Similar observations have been noted in Nigeria (Stock, 1983), India (Murthy, 1982), and Korea (Sich, 1981).

SOCIO-CULTURAL FACTORS

In some societies, pregnancy and child-bearing are still viewed as a natural process, so women may not use the formal health services for fear of interference from health workers. In India women were found not to be keen to seek preventive care, even if they were feeling unwell (Murthy, 1982). In Pakistan, women accepted illness before and after delivery as due to fate rather than due to human fault or negligence (Kazmi, 1991).

HEALTH AND ECONOMIC TRENDS IN ZAMBIA

The importance of all these factors in determining the utilization of health services has received considerable attention in both the United States and Britain, and has been the subject of a few studies in North and West Africa. There has been a lack of data on maternity services utilization in Zambia, however. The issue is particularly pertinent because Zambia introduced user fees for maternity care for the first time in 1993, a major change in orientation for a state which previously provided a free health service.

The fundamental changes in health care policy need to be understood within the changing economic conditions in Zambia. During the first decade after independence

	1983	1988	1990
Per capita income in real terms (US$)	660	250	175
Rates of inflation (%)	18	110	80
Budget of deficits [Zambian kwacha (K) million]	–	2194	2326

Figure 3.1 Adverse effects of Zambia's poor economic performance (Ministry of Health, Zambia, 1992).

(1964–1974), Zambia experienced rapid economic growth, averaging 7.9% per year. During this period employment expanded, and incomes increased accordingly. The government expanded educational facilities rapidly to meet the demand for skilled people. Health was also assigned a high priority and the health infrastructure developed quickly.

A rapid deterioration of the Zambian economy has occurred since 1974. Trends in per capita GNP showed a precipitous decline from just above US$700 in 1981 to US$250 in 1987, at constant prices, *Figure 3.1* (Bennett and Musambo, 1990).

A number of internal and external factors have been identified as contributing to the current economic crisis in Zambia. Among the internal factors, one of the most notable is the lack of diversification in the economy, with continued dependency on a single commodity, copper. Low market prices, combined with a subsequent fall in production, have led to considerable contraction of export earnings. The international impact of increases in oil prices and the unfavourable terms of trade for copper products resulted in a severe blow to the economy. It became increasingly necessary to borrow from abroad in order to finance imports (Bennett and Musambo, 1990).

Between 1983 and 1987, an International Monetary Fund (IMF)/World Bank-supported structural adjustment programme was initiated to redress the problems. However, the failure to arrest the decline in economic growth, combined with the negative social and political consequences of the adjustment measures, culminated in the government's suspension of the package. In 1988 an interim plan was designed and implemented by the government, independently of the IMF. The plan failed to control the money supply and a high rate of inflation resulted. Since January 1989 a series of radical monetary and fiscal policy measures have been introduced by the government with backing from the IMF and World Bank. These measures include devaluation of the national currency and monetary and fiscal restraint. Tax reform, public sector retrenchment, privatization of para-statals, and the phasing out of subsidies on maize meal and cooking oil have been implemented. These policies succeeded in reducing the fiscal deficit from 30% of GDP in 1986 to an estimated 8% in 1989.

HEALTH CARE FINANCING IN ZAMBIA

There are two main health care sectors in Zambia: the government sector and the non-government sector, which includes non-governmental organizations (NGOs) and the private sector. Government health services are financed mainly by revenue from general taxation. Part of the cost of non-governmental health services is met by patient fees.

In the past, government commitment to the financing of health care has been impressive, with approximately 8% of the budget going to the health sector. More recently, the health sector's share of expenditure has been eroded, particularly for capital expenditure; real per capita expenditure on the health sector declined by 50% between 1982 and 1987.

Initiatives for cost sharing

The policy of the government had been to provide health care free to all the people of Zambia, but in 1986 it accepted the IMF/World Bank conditions of user charges for most health services, with the exception of maternal and child health services. User charges were intended to generate funds at institutional level which could be used to meet local costs.

The government was reluctant to implement user fees at once, probably because of fear of the political repercussions from the public. An attempt to introduce user charges for health services in September 1987 was suspended due to a public outcry. Another attempt was made a year later. Only fees for prescriptions, medical examination, dental care, vaccinations for international travel, and in-patient care for non-Zambians were introduced at Lusaka's University Teaching Hospital and the central hospitals in the copper belt province. The nation-wide introduction of user fees in all health institutions, including maternity services, was effected in August 1993. Guidelines for implementation were worked out at the central level (Kawimbe and Katele, 1993).

In Lusaka, expectant mothers were required to pay 50 kwacha (K, exchange rate at October 1993: £1 = K560) for registration, K50 for each antenatal visit, K300 for a haemoglobin test, K600 for the Venereal Disease Reference Laboratory (VDRL) test, and K2500 for a delivery and postnatal care (Lusaka City Council, 1993). In addition to user charges, mothers were still required to buy two pairs of surgical gloves (K700), a packet of sanitary pads (K800), and a cord clamp (K350). In total, a mother had to spend approximately K1350 for antenatal care and K5600 for delivery. For a poor family household, whose monthly income is approximately K15,000 per month, expenditure on maternity care could account for a third of the monthly income.

STUDY OF THE DETERMINANTS OF MATERNITY SERVICE UTILIZATION IN A PERI-URBAN COMMUNITY

George Health Centre

George Health Centre lies approximately 7 km south-west of Lusaka and serves the largest peri-urban population of Lusaka. The 1990 census estimated the population of the George Health Centre catchment area to be 116,955 (Central Statistics Office, 1990). The population is engaged mainly in the informal sector, in activities such as carpentry and vegetable selling, but a substantial proportion is unemployed. Most people live in simple two- or three-roomed houses constructed from concrete blocks or mud bricks and roofed with corrugated asbestos, usually held down with stones. Each plot is approximately 10 m². Most homes have access to a pit latrine and there is a public standpipe of chlorinated water for every 25 houses.

Health services are provided by the government-run George Health Centre and by a private clinic. The government clinic was opened in 1982, initially providing curative services only. After 6 years, a maternal and child health (MCH) unit and labour ward were opened. George Health Centre provides 24 h delivery services, and antenatal clinic sessions are held five times a week. The clinic is linked to a radio communication system which is used to request transport for transferrals to the University Teaching Hospital. The labour ward is staffed by 17 midwives, who work shifts, while eight midwives are responsible for antenatal services.

The main objective of introducing these services was to try and bring them closer to the community. Mothers in this area are expected to utilize George Health Centre unless referred to the University Teaching Hospital for specialist obstetric care.

Objectives of the study

The specific objectives of the study were:

- To determine the effect of socio-demographic variables on the utilization of maternity services.
- To determine who are the principal decision-makers in the utilization of services.
- To analyse the effect of distance on utilization of services.
- To describe mothers' views of the maternity care services offered at George Health Centre.
- To determine the influence of traditional beliefs on utilization of services.
- To ascertain mothers' and midwives' attitudes to, and understanding of, user fees.
- To assess the immediate impact of user fees in the first few months of their introduction.

Methodology

Multiple methods of data collection were utilized including household interviews, focus-group discussions, examination of mothers' antenatal cards, and a review of clinic registers.

At the community and household levels, the purpose of the study was explained to the mothers prior to the interviews and focus-group discussions. Only mothers who were willing to participate in the study were included. Permission to conduct the study was obtained from the Ministry of Health, the Public Health Department of Lusaka City Council, and George Health Centre.

HOUSEHOLD INTERVIEWS

A total of 200 household interviews were conducted with mothers who had delivered a live baby between January and August 1993. The mothers were aged between 15 and 45 years. Recruitment was limited to women who had been residents of the study area for at least 5 years, who were well established in the community, and who would be expected to know about available health services. The sampling frame was the listings of compounds, census supervisory areas (CSAs), and supervisory enumeration areas (SEAs) taken from the Central Statistics Office (CSO).

A multi-stage cluster sampling method was employed. First, a list of all the compounds that fell into the George Health Centre catchment area was drawn up, from which six compounds were selected at random. Second, the CSAs in each of the selected compounds were listed and 15 CSAs selected randomly. From these a sample of 15 SEAs were selected randomly. Enumeration of all households in the chosen SEAs would have been the ideal, so as to perform a systematic sampling of the households. However, this was not possible due to logistical and time constraints. A 'snowball' sampling approach was adopted instead. Each successive interview was conducted with a relative or friend named by the previous interviewee. This method had the advantage that the interviewee had greater trust in the interviewer and therefore possibly supplied more accurate data. Selection bias may also have occurred, however.

Interviews took place in mothers' homes. The times were chosen to allow mothers to carry out their household chores, with an average duration for each interview of about 20 minutes. The interviews were conducted in Nyanja, which is the main local language in the area.

FOCUS-GROUP DISCUSSIONS

Three focus-group discussions were held. The first involved female community health workers, the second pregnant women, and the third the midwives at the health centre. The discussions covered the following areas:

- Timing of the first antenatal visit.
- Reasons why women prefer to deliver at home.
- Views on the services offered at the clinic.
- Perceptions towards the user fees.

Each focus group had a total of 10 participants, and discussions lasted about 45 minutes.

MOTHERS' ANTENATAL CARDS

The antenatal cards of the respondents in the household interviews were reviewed to elicit the following information:

- Gestation of pregnancy at booking.
- Number of antenatal visits.
- Blood tests and referrals.

HEALTH CENTRE REGISTERS

Registers at the MCH section and the labour ward of the George Health Centre for the period January 1990 to November 1994 were reviewed to examine the utilization patterns for antenatal and delivery care. For the purposes of this study 'antenatal attendance' was defined as at least one visit to the antenatal clinic during the most recent pregnancy.

Findings

CHARACTERISTICS OF THE HOUSEHOLD INTERVIEW SAMPLE

The age range, educational level, and marital status of the respondents are shown in *Figure 3.2.*

45

Age group	Percentage
15–19 years	22
20–24 years	37
25–29 years	25
30–34 years	9
35–39 years	3.5
40–44 years	3.5
Educational level	
Illiterate	13
Primary education	71
Secondary education	16
Marital status	
Married	89
Single	6
Separated	3
Divorced	2
Husband's employment	
Employed	70
Unemployed	30

Figure 3.2 Age range, educational level, marital status, and husband's employment for the household interview sample.

ANTENATAL CARE

A total of 86% of the women interviewed had received antenatal care during their most recent pregnancy. Of this group, 78% had attended George Health Centre during the second trimester of their pregnancy, while 7% attended during the third trimester; only 15% of the mothers booked during the first trimester. The advantage of starting antenatal care within the first 3 months of pregnancy is that a baseline assessment can be made, which makes early detection of any abnormalities easier. Essex and Everett (1977) showed that, in Tanzania, 80% of high-risk patients could be selected at the first antenatal visit.

THE DECISION-MAKING PROCESS

The observed high level of antenatal clinic attendance is similar to Zambia's national figure of 88% (Gaisie, 1992). The high level reflects the availability and easy accessibility of antenatal services in the George area. Of the women who obtained their care at health centres, 24 did so at centres other than George because they were employed in the formal sector and found it more convenient to attend clinics closer to their work places. Of the 14% who did not use the services, the largest group of non-attendees was among respondents who lived within 1 km of the health centre, suggesting that distance was not the primary deterrent.

Among the non-attendees, 69% said their husbands were unemployed and could not afford to buy the required items, such as baby layette, surgical gloves, and cord clamps. They reported that they were scared of being told off by the midwives. Distance was mentioned as a reason for non-attendance by 31%.

The majority (60%) of respondents said that 'feeling unwell' had prompted their decision to go to the antenatal clinic. Other reasons given were insufficient money to pay for the antenatal card (3%), and concern about the size of the pregnancy (10%).

Only 5% of the respondents said that they were advised to go by the nurse. During focus-group discussions, 80% of the participants confirmed that in the George area pregnant women generally only report early to the antenatal clinic if they are feeling unwell.

It seems that the antenatal clinic was viewed as a curative service for problems and complications. In a study carried out in a rural village in South East Botswana, 86.4% of women sought antenatal care in pregnancy; of these, three-quarters were motivated by a physical complaint (Ulin and Ulin, 1981).

Half of the respondents said that it was their personal decision to attend the antenatal clinic, 24% reported that their husband was the decision maker, while for 18% the decision was influenced by an elderly woman in the family (woman's own mother, mother-in-law, or grandmother).

CHILD CARE

Mothers were asked who looked after younger children and did the housework while they were at the antenatal clinic. Half of the respondents said that this was done by older children, 28% had help from an adult relative, 15% from their husband, and 7% from neighbours.

INFLUENCE OF TRADITIONAL PRACTICES ON ANTENATAL CLINIC ATTENDANCE

The focus-group participants gave some examples of the traditional practices which were carried out when a woman was expecting her first baby. Among the Bemba from the northern province, a woman expecting her first baby cannot go to the clinic until a female member of her husband's family has performed the traditional ceremony. This ceremony involves the smearing of cassava mealie-meal on the face and chest of the pregnant woman, and signifies to the public that the woman is pregnant. Among the Nyanja-speaking people from the eastern province, the pregnant woman is given a white cloth which she wears whenever she goes to the clinic. At a short ceremony, the pregnant woman is also given some money. Both of these ceremonies are held around the fifth month of pregnancy.

PLACE OF DELIVERY

The majority of compounds surveyed were located within 3 km of George Health Centre, so it would be expected that nearly all mothers would use the facility for birthing. However, this was not the case as 27% of the mothers who participated in the survey delivered at home (see *Figure 3.3*). Some of the reasons given were:

- "There was nobody to remain with the children at home."
- "Labour was quick."
- "There was no money to pay at the clinic."
- "I have always delivered my children at home."

Figure 3.3 Respondents' place of delivery.

Place of delivery	Number	Percentage
George Health Centre	101	51
University Teaching Hospital	26	13
Home	55	27
Other health facility	18	9
Total	**200**	**100**

When the focus-group participants discussed why some mothers chose not to deliver at the George Health Centre, the first reason given was lack of money. They further explained that mothers who deliver at home are either assisted by their neighbours or traditional birth attendants (TBAs). If problems arise following delivery, the woman is taken to the clinic.

In Africa the available data often show antenatal care coverage as being considerably higher than the coverage of institutional deliveries (Royston and Ferguson, 1985; Kwast, 1988). The Botswana study also showed that, while 86.4% of the women had sought antenatal care during pregnancy, only 30.7% chose to deliver in the village clinic (Ulin and Ulin, 1981).

The respondents who had delivered at the George Health Centre were asked to give reasons why they decided to have their babies there. Some said that the clinic was near to their homes and therefore convenient. Others felt they had little option, "I could not have gone anywhere else because we were informed by the midwives that we are all required to deliver at George clinic." According to health service policy mothers who live in the George Health Centre catchment area should not go to another clinic as they risk being sent away.

Mothers in the age groups often considered to be at higher risk of complications (15–19 years and 35–39 years) formed the highest percentage of home deliveries (15% and 31%, respectively), while 3% of home births were to mothers aged 40–44 years. These older mothers are at particular risk of obstetric complications.

ATTENDANT AT DELIVERY
A total of 80% of the survey respondents reported that a midwife attended their most recent birth, while 2% were assisted by doctors at the teaching hospital, 15% by relatives (mothers, grandmothers or sisters), 1% by a TBA, and 2% delivered by themselves.

MOTHERS' VIEWS ABOUT SERVICES AT THE GEORGE HEALTH CENTRE
The focus group participants said that generally they received good care from the midwives. They were quick to report, however, that a few midwives had a bad attitude to the patients: "If you call the midwife while in labour, the midwife slaps you and shouts at the patient saying, 'Don't call for our assistance, all we want is to find the baby already out'."

Participants identified other aspects of the clinic with which they were not satisfied: "After delivery, women are discharged without having a shower. So they go back home with dry blood on their legs". "Even the baby is not bathed". "Following delivery, women are not given tea or porridge. Women who deliver at night have to wait for their relatives to bring some food the following morning". "We cannot use the toilet because it is always locked".

Half the respondents in the household interviews and 80% in the focus-group discussions cited failure to provide food following delivery and not being able to have a bath as service factors with which they were unhappy.

One participant described an encounter with the security guard at the health centre: "I went to the clinic with my husband when labour started. On arrival, we knocked and the security guard asked if my husband had brought a bucket of water, even before he opened the gate for us. My husband replied 'No, how can I when I have no relative to draw the water?'. The security guard then asked my husband to go back and bring the water, while I was asked to lie on a bench, where I delivered without any assistance."

The process of labour is a critical time in a woman's life. Women during this time prefer to be in an environment in which people care. A home delivery is a favourite option for many women, because both psychological and emotional needs are met by relatives and friends. These aspects appeared to be lacking at the George Health Centre.

The important role of quality of care as a key determinant in health services' utilization has been emphasized by several authors (Lasker, 1981; Stock, 1983). Some of the deficiencies cited in the provision of maternity care may have accounted for some women opting for alternative care in institutions located several kilometres from their area of residence. Some respondents chose to travel up to 8 km to deliver their babies at the University Teaching Hospital. These women paid K30,000 in comparison to K2500, which is the fee at the George Health Centre. When asked why they did not use the George Health Centre for delivery, the women said that they wanted 'better care'. They were able to make this choice as they were of a higher socioeconomic status and were employed in the formal sector.

Women in the household survey reported that they were willing to wait up to 2 h at the antenatal clinic. The focus-group participants said that the waiting time at the antenatal clinic was too long, however. "We report at the clinic at 5 o'clock and the clinic only opens at 8 o'clock. Even then the nurses do not start seeing the patients there and then. They first of all chat among themselves. Therefore, most often, the earliest time we leave the clinic is around 10.30 or 11.30."

USER FEES AND THEIR EFFECTS
The users' views

The majority of participants in the focus groups and 80% of the respondents in the household interviews reported that they did not know why user fees had been introduced: "All we saw was that from 1st August, we were required to pay for health services. And we wonder, before fee paying was introduced, we were required to buy gloves, pads and pegs [cord clamps]. We thought since we now have to pay user fees, there is now no need to buy these items."

They ventured the following possible reasons:

• "Maybe to buy drugs since we are told there are no drugs at the clinic."

• "To raise money to pay health workers."

• "The government is now going into business."

It is sometimes argued that user fees for government health services are merely an extension of the practice of paying traditional healers, and should therefore not cause undue problems. The participants were asked about this:

> *Consulting the traditional healers has always been there. When modern medicine fails, people usually opt to see the traditional healer whose fees are usually affordable, and terms of payment are suitable; for example, one can pay the money in instalments. To raise the money, relatives usually contribute towards the fee. In fact, we see the traditional healer as being in business. We are therefore surprised that the government is going into business too. We thought the government is there to protect the poor.*

The respondents of the household interviews reported that a K50 fee for each antenatal visit was fine and they could pay. However, a common complaint was that the fee for blood tests was too expensive. A review of mothers' antenatal cards showed that the majority of the mothers (90%) did not have a haemoglobin or VDRL test done. One woman said that she attended the antenatal clinic only once because she was afraid to go back, as she had been told to have blood tests done, but could not afford them.

Of the household survey respondents, 60% said that they could afford the user fees that had been introduced. However, the focus-group participants were less optimistic, saying that most of them could not afford the fees. The problem was with the K2500 required for delivery care. They felt that the government should consider reducing the fee to K500 or devise means of exempting poor people. When asked why women cannot save money for the delivery, the focus group participants replied: "Even if we save, we give priority to buying food."

Of the mothers who had home deliveries, 12% explained that they could not afford to raise the delivery fee. Some of these respondents (6%) had no source of income because their husbands were unemployed. During the household interviews it was observed that such families depended on their parents for support. When user fees have been implemented, clients from low socioeconomic groups appear to be more affected than those who are better off.

Midwives' views about user fees

The midwives had a different perspective from the user group. They were all of the opinion that the introduction of user fees was a step towards meeting some of the requirements of the health service. They explained that, in the long term, a few items, such as patients' food, should be purchased to help ease the shortage of resources. They pointed out that the current fee of K50 for antenatal care was too little to contribute to improving services, and advocated an increase in fees.

Effect of user fees on clinic use for pregnancy and delivery care

Health centre records revealed that there was a reduction in the number of new antenatal attendees (see *Figure 3.4*) and of repeat visits during the first 6 months following the introduction of user fees. During the household interviews, approximately 10% of the respondents said that they did not use the George Health Centre for delivery because they could not afford the delivery fee. This was reiterated in the focus-group discussions.

In the month of July 1993, the clinic conducted 282 deliveries, but this figure fell to 233 at the end of August after charges had been introduced. *Figure 3.5* shows the pattern of deliveries at the George Health Centre since 1990. A decline in health centre deliveries is observable during the last two quarters of 1993, with the monthly number of deliveries decreasing by about 11%. This scenario gradually reverted to normal, and in the last quarter of 1994 attendance rates and the number of clinic deliveries compare more favourably with those of the pre user-fee period. Perhaps by then the mothers in the George area had accepted the user fees as inevitable.

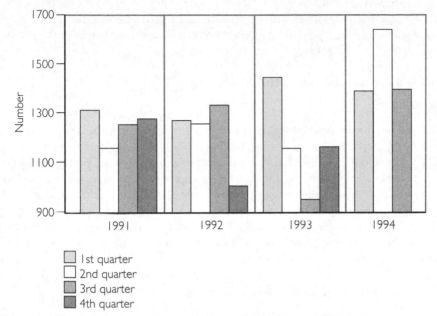

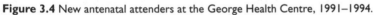

□ 1st quarter
□ 2nd quarter
■ 3rd quarter
■ 4th quarter

Figure 3.4 New antenatal attenders at the George Health Centre, 1991–1994.

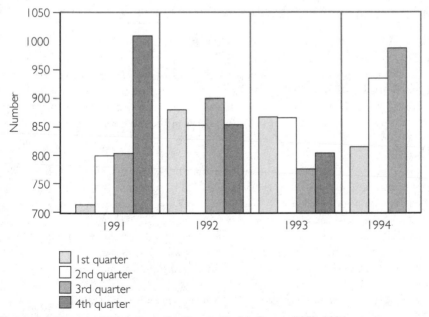

□ 1st quarter
□ 2nd quarter
■ 3rd quarter
■ 4th quarter

Figure 3.5 Pattern of deliveries at the George Health Centre, 1991–1994.

Conclusions from the study

A number of factors that appear to play an important role in the uptake of maternity services in the George area were identified. The most important ones centre on the quality of services and their cost.

Recommendations from the study

MIDWIFERY PRACTICE

- A dialogue should be established between the midwives and the women in the community through the existing communication channels (e.g., female community health workers). This is essential for two-way education to take place. Midwives need to be educated regarding mothers' feelings about current services, while women need to be educated about the importance of using antenatal services early in pregnancy and the need for supervised delivery by a trained person.
- Midwives should consider allowing relatives to come to the health centre to stay with the mother during labour. This will help meet the mothers' emotional needs and make the services more acceptable.
- To reduce the current long waiting time at the antenatal clinic, a two-shift system could be introduced so that all mothers do not arrive at the same time.

RESEARCH

The impact on antenatal and delivery attendance rates needs to be monitored carefully at all health facilities where fees are introduced or where fees are significantly increased. Further data may have to be collected to ascertain whether any delay in seeking care occurs because of difficulty in raising the money for the fees

DEVELOPMENT OF A CLEAR POLICY TOWARDS THE PROTECTION OF THOSE UNABLE TO AFFORD USER CHARGES

Midwives, with the collaboration of TBAs and community health workers in the area, need to identify those women who are most in need and make some arrangements to assist them. This might be through the Ministry of Community Development and Social Welfare, or through the use of a sliding scale of fees to cater for the poor.

REFERENCES

Abbas, A.A. and Walker, G.J.A. (1986) Determinants of the utilization of maternal and child health services in Jordan. *International Journal of Epidemiology*, **15**(3): 404–407.

Airey, T. (1989) The impact of road construction on hospital in-patient catchments in the Meru District of Kenya. *Social Science and Medicine*, **29**(1): 95–106.

Andersen, R. and Newman, J.F. (1973). Societal and individual determinants of medical care utilization in the United States. *Milbank Memorial Fund Quarterly*, **51**: 95–124

Annis, S. (1981) Physical access and utilization of health services in rural Guatemala. *Social Science and Medicine*, **15**(D): 515–523.

Bennett, S. and Musambo, M. (1990) *Report on Community Financing and District Management Strengthening in Zambia*. UNICEF, New York.

Benyoussef, A. and Wessen, F.A. (1974) Utilization of health services in developing countries – Tunisia. *Social Science and Medicine*, **8**(5): 287–304.

Buekens, P. (1990) Variations in provision and uptake of antenatal care. *Bailliere's Clinical Obstetrics and Gynaecology*, **4**(1): 187–203.

Central Statistics Office (1990) *Census of Population, Housing and Agriculture*. Central Statistics Office, Lusaka.

Dia, A. (1990) Maternal mortality in Senegal: Contributing factors in the health system and the community. Draft Report. In: Thaddeus, S. and Maine, D. (eds), *Too Far To Walk: Maternal Mortality in Context. Findings From A Multidisciplinary Literature Review*. Prevention of Maternal Mortality Program, Center for Population and Family Health, Columbia University School of Public Health, Columbia.

Dor, A. and Gaag, J. (1988) *The Demand for Medical Care in Developing Countries – Quantity Rationing in Rural Cote d'Ivoire*. Living Standards Measurement Study (LSMS) Working Paper No. 35, World Bank, Washington, DC.

Egunjobi, L. (1983) Factors influencing choice of hospitals: A case study of the northern part of Oyo State, Nigeria. *Social Science and Medicine*, **17**(9): 585–589.

Essex, B.J. and Everett, V.J. (1977) Use of action oriented record card for antenatal screening. *Tropical Doctor*, **7**: 134–138.

Frank, R.G. (1990) Hospital ownership and the care of uninsured and medicaid patients: Findings from the National Hospital Survey 1979–1984. *Health Policy*, **14**: 1–11.

Freeman, D.H. (1983) A categorical analysis of contacts in the family health clinic, Calabar, Nigeria. *Social Science and Medicine*, **17**(9): 571–578.

Gaisie, K. (1992) *Zambia Demographic and Health Survey*. University of Zambia, Lusaka, Central Statistical Office, Lusaka, and Macro International Inc., Columbia, Maryland.

Graham, W.J. and Campbell, O. (1990) *Measuring Maternal Health: Defining the Issues*. Maternal and Child Epidemiology Unit, London School of Hygiene and Tropical Medicine, London.

Habib, O.S. and Vaughan, J.P. (1986) The determinants of health services utilization in Southern Iraq: A household interview survey. *International Journal of Epidemiology*, **15**(3): 395–403.

Hickey, M.U. and Kasonde, J.M. (1977) Maternal mortality at University Teaching Hospital, Lusaka. *Medical Journal of Zambia*, **11**(13): 74–78.

Jolly, R. and King, M. (1966) *Medical Care in Developing Countries*. Oxford University Press, Oxford.

Kawimbe, B. and Katele, K. (1993) *Paying For Quality Health Care (Community Co-Financing: Mwanse–Mphangwe Initiative)*. Health Reforms Implementation Guidelines Hand Book (2), Ministry of Health, Lusaka.

Kazmi, S. (1991) *Safe Motherhood Consumer View Points, Sample Survey*. Marketing and Research Consultants (MARC), Association of Business Professional and Agricultural Women, Pakistan (unpublished).

Kohn, R. and White, K. (eds) (1976) *Health Care: An International Collaborative Study of Medical Utilization*. WHO, Geneva.

Kloos, H. (1987) Illness and behaviour in Addis Ababa and rural central Ethiopia. *Social Science and Medicine*, **25**(9): 1003–1019.

Kwast, B.E. (1988) Factors associated with maternal mortality in Addis Ababa, Ethiopia. *International Journal of Gynaecology and Obstetrics*, **17**(1): 115–121.

Kwast, B.E. (1989) Maternal mortality: Levels, causes and promising interventions. *Journal of Biosocial Science*, **10**: 51–67.

Lasker, R.J.N. (1981) Choosing among therapies: Illness behaviour in the Ivory Coast. *Social Science and Medicine* **15**(A): 157–168

Lusaka City Council (1993) *Revised Cost Sharing Scheme in Lusaka Urban Clinics*. Public Health Department, Lusaka.

Mahler, H. (1987) The safe motherhood initiative: A call to action. *The Lancet*, **I**(8534): 668–670.

Mhango, C. (1986) Reproductive mortality in Lusaka, Zambia. *Studies in Family Planning*, **17**(5): 243–251.

Ministry of Health, Zambia (1992) *Health Reforms in Zambia*. Ministry of Health, Zambia, Lusaka.

Murthy, N. (1982) Reluctant patients – the women of India. *World Health Forum*, **3**: 315–316.

Nnadi, E.E. and Kabat, H.F. (1984) Choosing health care services in Nigeria: A developing nation. *Journal of Tropical Medicine and Hygiene*, **87**: 47–51.

Orubuloye, I.O. and Caldwell, J.C. (1975) The impact of public health services on mortality: A study of mortality differentials in a rural area of Nigeria. *Population Studies*, **29**(2): 259–272.

Pinot, J.A. and Faundes, A. (1989) Obstetric and gynaecological care for third world women. *International Journal of Gynaecology and Obstetrics*, **21**: 361–369.

Poole, D.L. and Carlton, T.O. (1986) A model for analysing utilization of maternal and child health services. *Health and Social Work*, **1**(3): 209–222.

Population Reports (1988) *Mothers' Lives Matter: Maternal Health in the Community*. Series 1,7, Johns Hopkins University, Baltimore.

Ray, S.K. (1984) Extent of utilization of maternal care services of PHC by the families of a rural area. *Indian Journal of Public Health*, **3**: 122–127.

Reid, M.E. and Macilwaine, D.M. (1980) Consumer opinion of a hospital antenatal clinic. *Social Science and Medicine*, **14**(A): 363–368.

Rooney, C. (1992) *Antenatal Care and Maternal Health: How Effective Is It? A review of the evidence*. WHO, Geneva.

Royston, E. and Ferguson, J. (1985) The coverage of maternity care: A critical review of available information. *World Health Statistics*, **38**: 267–273.

Sich, D. (1981) Traditional concepts and customs in pregnancy, birth and postpartum period in rural Korea. In: Thaddeus, S. and Maine, D. (eds), *Too Far To Walk: Maternal Mortality in Context. Findings From A Multidisciplinary Literature Review*. Prevention of Maternal Mortality Program, Center for Population and Family Health, Columbia University School of Public Health, Columbia.

Simpson, H. and Walker, G. (1980) When do pregnant women attend for antenatal care? *British Medical Journal*, **11**: 104–187.

Stock, R. (1983) Distance and the utilization of health facilities in rural Nigeria. *Social Science and Medicine*, **17**(9): 563–570.

Tew, M. (1990) *Safer Childbirth? A Critical History of Maternity Care*. Chapman & Hall, London.

Thaddeus, S. and Maine, D. (1990) *Too Far To Walk: Maternal Mortality In Context. Findings from a Multidisciplinary Literature Review*. Prevention of Maternal Mortality Program, Center for Population and Family Health, Columbia University School of Public Health, Columbia.

Ulin, R.U. and Ulin, O.U. (1981) The use and non-use of preventive health services in a Southern Africa village. *International Journal of Health Education*, **4**: 45–53.

Voorhoeve, A.M. (1982) Modern and traditional antenatal and delivery care. In: Van Ginneken, J.K. and Muller, A.S. (eds), *Maternal and Child Health in Rural Kenya*. Croom Helm, London and Sydney, pp 309–322.

WHO (1986) Maternal mortality: Helping women off the road to death. *WHO Chronicle*, **40**(5): 175–183.

Wong, E.L. (1987) Accessibility, quality of care and prenatal care in the Philippines. *Social Science and Medicine*, **24**: 927–944.

Young, J.C. (1981) Non-use of physicians: methodological approaches, policy implications, and the utility of decision models. *Social Science and Medicine*, **15**(B): 499–507.

The Costs of 'Adjustment': User Charges for Maternity Care

Susan F. Murray

Much of the discussion within the Safe Motherhood Initiative has centred on how to improve access to maternity care. It has become clear that for many women in many countries there are substantial barriers to receiving timely and adequate care, particularly in emergency situations. It is argued convincingly that access could be improved through the provision of essential obstetric functions at first referral level (WHO, 1991), through the construction of maternity waiting homes near hospitals (Farnot Carduso, 1986; Poovan *et al.*, 1990), and so on. However, there is a major access issue which has not as yet featured greatly in the Safe Motherhood discussions, and which may directly militate against these innovations. It is a trend with increasing significance in the world scene – the charging of fees for the use of maternity services.

In the past few years user charges for government health services have been introduced or increased substantially in many countries. The background to this was the drastic economic decline which took place in many developing countries, being most acute in Africa. In the 1980s there was a massive decline in world prices for the primary commodities on which the continent depends. The quality of the health services in many countries has deteriorated dramatically as a result. Foreign exchange to purchase drugs and other imported medical supplies has become increasingly scarce. On top of this, the AIDS pandemic has overwhelmed the meagre capacity of many countries' health facilities.

The spiral of debt compounds their problems. Sub-Saharan Africa, the world's poorest region, repays its creditors US$10 billion each year in debt servicing, four times as much as governments spend on the health and education of their citizens (Oxfam, 1993). This amount represents only a third of what is actually due, and arrears are building up. Restraints on government spending, especially on social programmes, have been reinforced by loan conditions imposed by the International Monetary Fund (IMF) and the World Bank. Structural adjustment programmes usually involve some combination of curtailment of government expenditure, currency devaluation, trade liberalization (with removal of government subsidies), and price controls, and a general reorientation of the economy towards the generation of more foreign exchange, both through import reduction and export promotion. These are a requirement in return for further loans. According to the IMF and the World Bank, these adjustment packages will lead to economic growth and ultimately poverty reduction. However, the immediate results of structural adjustment programmes for the poor are usually rapid price rises for food and transport, and the introduction of school and medical fees. At the same time, wages fall and unemployment increases.

With increasing pressure being brought to bear on economies for debt repayment, government expenditure on health and education is squeezed even further. There results a migration of skilled health workers, and private practice spreads.

MINIMUM PACKAGES OF CARE

Recently, considerable work has been done at a theoretical level to define what might be the minimal acceptable levels of health service provision (WHO, 1984; World Bank, 1993). In its World Development Report, *Investing in Health,* the World Bank advocated that governments supply 'a well-defined package of essential services'. This package of public health and clinical services is costed at US$12 per capita per annum for low income countries and at US$20 for the middle income countries. Out of this amount, the minimum *clinical* package would cost US$4 in low income countries and US$7.5 in middle income countries, half of these amounts (US$2 and £3.5, respectively) being for antenatal and delivery care.

However, it is highly debatable whether even this minimum package is realistic for those countries in which there has already been the almost complete collapse of government revenues for welfare services. Government expenditure on health in Uganda is US$1.4 per capita yearly – a decline in real terms of 95% since 1972 and it is only US$0.53 per capita in Zaire (Poore, 1993). As Peter Poore of Save the Children Fund has pointed out, no-one can reallocate, or better manage, funds that do not exist.

The World Bank acknowledges that the prospects for health services are pretty bleak, and has encouraged two strategies as a result. First, it has tried to persuade donors to target their aid to the health services, but this has had limited success. The changes in Eastern Europe have actually channelled donor aid away from Africa, and levels of foreign aid to developing countries actually decreased during the 1980s. British aid, for example, was reduced in real terms from £2 billion in 1979 to just under 1.6 billion by the end of the 1980s (Editorial, 1990). Second, the World Bank advocates a greater role for the private sector in the delivery of health care, to run alongside 'raised efficiency' in the public sector, part financed by fee-for-service arrangements.

FEES FOR SERVICES

The 'fee for service' element of the World Bank strategy – user charges – may have profound implications for maternity health services, and it merits our close attention. User fees are sometimes advocated as a means of reducing the 'frivolous' use of services (although there is very little evidence to support this), and they are often advocated as a means of cost recovery, either for the basic service requirements, such as drugs, or in order to provide improved quality of care.

Charles Griffin, an economist who authored the World Bank seminar paper *User Charges for Health Care in Principle and Practice* (Griffin, 1988), has suggested the following 'working hypothesis' to justify charging for care. He predicts that there will be some negative effects for those people already using government services. These will take the form of a reduced probability of seeking care from government services and of smaller quantities being purchased, but he argues that these effects will be quite weak. On the plus side, if the quantity of care supplied is currently being constrained by the lack of funding the service receives, then the small negative effect of a price increase on use should, he argues, be outweighed by the increased service available for those who are currently unable to obtain government services at all. Griffin also suggests that there may be other desirable outcomes, because higher revenues would allow governments to expand certain areas of care. More might be spent by the government on public health interventions, for example, if the burden of curative services on their budgets is reduced.

What is questionable in the current context of declining purchasing power, is whether user charges can actually generate sufficient revenue to finance health service improvements or expansion in care. It is estimated that the most that such cost recovery measures can raise, when the system is well-established and functioning to capacity, will be 5–10% of recurrent costs. But even then, as Gilson and Russell (1994) point out, there are many ways of measuring both fees and costs. The 'on-the-ground' experiences of fee introduction have often been highly problematic.

In Tanzania charges for maternity hospital services were introduced at the beginning of 1994, and facilities were then, in theory at least, provided according to three grades. The cheapest, Grade 3, involved an initial one-off fee of 800 TSh (about £1.00; TSh = TShillings), for consultation and admission, the rest then being free. Grade 1 patients, on the other hand, were to be charged for each item of care separately – 600 TSh for a normal delivery, 600 TSh for haemoglobin, 2000 TSh a day for bed occupancy in a single or two-bedded room, 15,000 TSh for a caesarean section, and even 4000 TSh for an episiotomy!

Women opted for the grade they preferred and could afford, and 98% of patients at the regional referral hospital I visited in March 1994 had opted for the cheapest, Grade 3. This was something which came as no surprise when one walked around the unit for, apart from having marginally more privacy, the higher grade patients had no better facilities than anyone else, the same broken bedsteads, torn mattresses and curtainless windows. The end result was that all the Grade 1 and 2 rooms were empty at the time of my visit, all the women were crowded into a smaller space than previously, hospital admissions were reported as being down, and 15,000–20,000 TSh was being collected per day. This was not going to make any huge inroads into cost recovery, given that the cost of a pair of gloves was 1000 TSh and an intravenous infusion was 2000–3000 TSh. It all hardly seemed worth the increased administration involved.

IS IT POSSIBLE TO GENERALIZE FROM SMALL PROJECTS?
There are certainly instances, many of these from the Bamako Initiative, in which the introduction of user fees seems to have been successful in the local community co-financing of health services. The danger is in generalizing the successful experience

of a small project (which often has seed money to provide an initial improvement in services or supplies) to national government programmes (which usually do not). In a suburb of Dakar in Senegal, for example, there was a notably successful community financing scheme for primary health care, which charged consultation fees and payment for essential drugs. However, when this was generalized from an urban population to the whole country, the model failed (Fassin and Gentlini, 1989). Rural communities were less well-off than city dwellers and less committed politically to the idea than the community in the pilot project area had been. The underprivileged actually became worse off because the policy officially disengaged the Ministry of Public Health from remote areas.

This raises the issue which must be of most concern – the impact of user charges on the poorest people. Some work has been done in this field. Gertler and van der Gaag (1990) suggested that a modest rise in health service charges is likely to reduce the use of services substantially for those on a very low income, while those whose needs are least will continue to use the services. In Swaziland, charges for government health services led to a big shift towards the use of mission services (which were already charging fees). More importantly, there was an overall drop in the use of formal health services of 17%, with a disproportionate drop in their use by low income households (Yoder, 1989).

EXEMPTION SYSTEMS

Most advocates of fees for service agree that there should be some way of exempting the poorest from paying the fees. This is not simple to resolve in practice. 'Willingness' and 'ability' to pay are not necessarily simple to define. One might, for example, use land ownership as an important indicator of ability to pay, but even then, as Korte *et al.* (1992) have pointed out, the cost of treatment for a family member constitutes one of the primary reasons for peasants *selling* their land in Bangladesh and Thailand. In some contexts paying for health care treatment may be the beginning of a downward spiral that removes a family's source of security and livelihood for the future.

There are two types of targeting the poor that can be used (Russell and Gilson, 1995). Characteristic targeting provides benefits to all the people with a given characteristic; for example, everyone in a certain age group, living in a particular geographic area, or with a specific health condition. Direct-targeting exemption systems, on the other hand, try to identify specific individuals or households according to their income status. In theory, this is more accurate in discriminating between the poor and the non-poor, but in the real world, where health services infrastructures are far from strong, the system may be underfunded, poorly administered, and arbitrary (Lennock, 1994). In Zimbabwe, for example, fee exemption requires assessment by the Social Welfare Officer. The nearest administrative office may be some 40–50 km away, and the bus fare costs more than the fee for registering at the health centre or hospital (Lennock, 1994). This sort of situation results in under-coverage of those patients who are actually eligible for free or reduced cost services. In other situations, the problem may be that there is leakage of subsidies to people who can actually afford to pay, but who have a special relationship with the persons taking the decision (Russell and Gilson, 1995).

LEVEL OF FEES

As is shown in Esnart Namakando's Zambian study (Chapter 3, this volume), the level at which the fees are set is likely to have significant impact on the timely uptake of services. The potential users' ease of access to cash will also be important. This varies from community to community, depending on how each economy is organized. An example from the Adamaoua province of Cameroon is often cited by advocates of user fees to show how these can successfully improve quality of service, while not deterring the poorer sectors of the community. However, this province's grasslands and cattle-raising tradition mean that cash is obtainable through sale of livestock when required (Litvack and Bodart, 1993). Not all communities can raise cash easily and, more particularly, not all women have access to, or control over, any money available.

It is also sometimes argued that people in Africa and elsewhere are accustomed to paying traditional healers and TBAs for their services, the implication being that they can equally well afford fees for formal health services (Ofosu-Amaah, 1989). However, this analogy is superficial. The form and conditions of payment in the non-formal sector are often more flexible. Payments are not always required immediately or in one go, they may be made in kind (that is, in goods or services rather than in cash), and they are normally set with the knowledge of the family's circumstances. It is very rare for health staff in the formal sector to be able to modify their fee system in such a flexible manner.

The introduction of health service charges may be exacerbated by the already existing 'second economy in health' in many countries. 'Free' health services are not always as free as they seem. It is quite well-known that some government health workers in Uganda (Van der Heijden, 1992), Tanzania (Abel-Smith and Rawal, 1992), and many other countries have developed a range of what might be termed 'economic survival strategies' to supplement their token, often delayed, salaries. Informally charging patients for nominally free services seems to be one of the commonest strategies. (Health service drugs and equipment ending up in the market place is another such strategy.) Unless health workers' salaries and conditions improve, informal charging is unlikely to cease. Service users then face two sets of 'fees' to pay.

USER FEES FOR REPRODUCTIVE HEALTH SERVICES

If we turn now to look specifically at reproductive health care, it is apparent that there is a trend to introduce charges for family planning services (Johns Hopkins University, 1991), and for services for the treatment and prevention of communicable diseases. The little evidence that exists suggest that such policy changes may have quite serious consequences.

A study by Stephen Moses et al. (1992) looked at the impact of a short-lived policy of charging fees to patients on attendance at a referral centre for sexually transmitted diseases (STDs) in Nairobi. They showed that when user fees approximately equivalent to half a day's wages were introduced, the seasonally adjusted mean monthly attendance by men reduced significantly – to 40% of its former level – and the attendance by women reduced to 65%. The introduction of user fees probably increased the number of untreated STDs in the population, with potentially serious long-term health implications. Price increases of around 60% for contraceptives in Bangladesh's social marketing project in 1990 had an immediate and severe effect on condom sales, with sales for the following 12 months down by nearly 50%. The effect on oral contraceptives was less dramatic – sales in the year following dropped slightly. Previously, however, sales had been rising rapidly each year (Cizewiski and Harvey, 1994).

USER FEES FOR MATERNITY SERVICES

There is remarkably little information available on the specific effect of user fees on the uptake of maternity services, and almost no published information on the effect such cost-recovery methods might have on quality of maternity care services. The fragmentary picture that we have so far, however, affords little ground for complacency.

In Zaire, first-time antenatal visits fell from 95% to 84% when the user fees increased abruptly in price in 1986 from 6 'egg equivalents' to 9 'egg equivalents' – the price of eggs in the local market (De Bethune *et al.*, 1989). In Ghana there was a major increase in fees for most health services in 1985 (maternity care exempted), and a sharp drop in the use of clinics followed. Urban clinic attendance gradually returned to the pre-1985 level, but the drop in rural utilization was sustained. Then, in 1988, mothers were asked to pay for delivery and for all drugs that were prescribed. The routine statistics from Komfo Anokye Teaching Hospital, Kumasi, show how the number of admissions to the maternity block dropped from 14,700 in 1987 to 13,187 in 1988, and how deliveries in the unit fell from 10,711 to 9447, returning to near the previous levels a year later (Martey *et al.*, 1993).

In Zimbabwe, whose health service was once the finest in Africa, the health budget for 1993–1994 was the lowest in real terms since independence. It had fallen by 36% over the previous 3 years (Africa Health Newsdesk, 1994). One result has been the continued increase in user fees, which has been the subject of much criticism from political figures, civil rights groups, and NGOs. The number of babies 'born before arrival' and later requiring admission to the Harare Central Hospital increased by one-third in the 6 months following stricter enforcement of charges in June 1991 (Logie and Woodroffe, 1993). Lennock (1994) reports that mortality among these babies rose by 156% in the same period, and that surveys in January 1993 confirmed that one of the major reasons for giving birth at home was the cost of delivery at health facilities. According to UNICEF figures, maternal mortality in Zimbabwe rose from 101 maternal deaths per 100,000 live births in 1989 to 350 per 100,000 live births in 1992. The direct relationship of this rise to the health services' economic circumstances is complicated by the rise in maternal death from AIDS during the same period, but what is clear is that the services, and its potential users, are under great pressure.

In Nigeria, where the government introduced a structural adjustment programme after oil prices slumped in the mid-1980s, data covering the most recent decade have shown a drastic decline in hospital births in university teaching hospitals throughout the country, and an increase in the incidence of maternal deaths in hospital (Tahzib, 1990). Owa *et al.* (1992) reviewed the effect of user charges on the use of maternity services and perinatal health in the Wesley Guild Hospital, Ilesha, where they were introduced in late 1984. They noted 'a striking and sustained decline' in attendances for antenatal care and for delivery at the hospital. Since more high-risk mothers were delivering at home, the pattern of admissions to the neonatal unit also changed. During 1981–1983 (pre-fees), 48% of admissions were babies born outside of hospital, but by 1987–1990 this had risen to 66% of admissions. The hospital perinatal mortality rate also rose, with many babies being brought in with birth asphyxia, umbilical infection or jaundice, and tetanus. More pre-term babies were also being admitted after being born outside the hospital, many of them with very low core temperatures.

At Ahmadu Bello University Teaching Hospital, Zaria, the number of obstetric admissions declined from 7450 per year in 1983 (when all aspects of maternity care in the hospital were free) to 5437 2 years later, when fees for some services were introduced, and to 3376 in 1988, by which time patients were being asked to pay for most of the materials needed for their treatment (Ekwempu *et al.*, 1990). The maternal deaths in the hospital rose by 56% between 1985 and 1988. The reasons for this have been debated, but probably include deterioration of the hospital services due to lack of funding, and delay in the decision to use hospital services because of increased fees. Most patients only came to hospital as a last resort once a complication had developed, and even then a long time was spent by relatives searching around for money or materials. Also, the mean interval between admission and surgery had increased strikingly.

The evidence is far from complete. What we know so far suggests that the introduction of, or increase in, user fees in many contexts has presented barriers to women requiring timely access to maternity care. Charges for contraceptives and for other reproductive health services may also put women's health at greater risk. This area remains under-researched, yet it may affect profoundly the work and the effectiveness of midwives in many countries. It should be the concern of health care providers everywhere, and the work begun by Namakando (see Chapter 3) to document the impact of the introduction of user fees in Zambia needs to be extended and be replicated by midwives in many countries. Only then will we know if the impact of fees for maternity care is regressive (as I am suggesting above) or progressive (as the World Bank would like it to be). Only in this way, too, may we avoid the risk of an ever-widening gap between the rhetoric of the safe motherhood theory, and the reality of practice in a time of economic crisis.

REFERENCES

Abel-Smith, B. and Rawal, P. (1992) Can the poor afford 'free' health services? A case study of Tanzania. *Health Policy and Planning,* **7**(9): 329–341.

Africa Health Newsdesk (1994) Zimbabwe: Crisis; what crisis? *Africa Health,* **March**: 6.

Cizewiski, R.L. and Harvey, P.D. (1994) The effect of price increases on contraceptive sales in Bangladesh. *Journal of Biosocial Science,* **26**: 25–35.

De Bethune, X., Alfani, S. and Lahaye, J.P. (1989) The influence of an abrupt price increase on health service utilisation: Evidence from Zaire. *Health Policy and Planning,* **4**: 76–81.

Editorial (1990) Structural adjustment and health in Africa. *Lancet,* **335**: 885–886.

Ekwempu, C.C., Maine, D., Olorukoba, M.B., Essien, E.S., and Kisseika, M.N. (1990) Structural adjustment and health in Africa. *Lancet,* **336**(8703): 56–57.

Farnot Carduso, U. (1986) Giving birth is safe now. *World Health Forum,* **7**: 348–352.

Fassin, D. and Gentlini, M. (1989) Letter. *Lancet,* **1**(8630): 162–163.

Gertler, P. and van der Gaag, J. (1990) *The Willingness to Pay for Medical Care: Evidence from Two Developing Countries.* World Bank, Washington DC.

Gilson, L. and Russell, S. (1994) Can fees recover costs? *Health Action,* **9**: 9.

Griffin, C.C. (1988) *User Charges for Health Care in Principle and Practice.* Economic Development Institute Seminar Paper No 37, World Bank, Washington DC.

Johns Hopkins University (1991) *Paying for Family Planning.* Population Reports Series J, No 39, Johns Hopkins University, Baltimore.

Korte, R., Richter, H., Merkle, F., and Gorgen, H. (1992) Financing health services in Sub-Saharan Africa: Options for decision makers during adjustment. *Social Science and Medicine,* **34**(1): 1–9.

Lennock, J. (1994) *Paying for Health: Poverty and Structural Adjustment in Zimbabwe.* Oxfam, Oxford.

Litvack, J.I. and Bodart, C. (1993) User fees plus quality equals improved access to health care. *Social Science and Medicine,* **37**(3): 369–383.

Logie, D.E. and Woodroffe, J. (1993) Structural adjustment: The wrong prescription for Africa? *British Medical Journal,* **307**: 41–44.

Martey, J.O., Djan, J.O., Twum, S., Browne, E.N.L., and Opoku, S.A. (1993) Maternal mortality due to haemorrhage in Ghana. *International Journal of Gynaecology and Obstetrics,* **42**(3): 237–242.

Moses, S., Manji, F., Bradley, J.E., Nagelkerke, N.J., Malisa, M.A., and Plummer, F.A. (1992) Impact of user fees on attendance at a referral centre for sexually transmitted diseases in Kenya. *Lancet,* **340**: 463–466.

Ofosu-Amaah, S. (1989) The Bamako Initiative. *Lancet,* **1**(8630): 162.

Owa, J.A., Osinaike, A.I., and Costello, A.M. de L. (1992) Charging for health services in developing countries. *Lancet,* **340**: 732.

Oxfam (1993) *Africa, Make or Break.* Oxfam, Oxford.

Poore, P. (1993) World Bank's World Development Report (letter). *Lancet,* **342**: 44.

Poovan, P., Kifle, F., and Kwast, B.E. (1990) A maternity waiting home reduces obstetric catastrophes. *World Health Forum,* **11**: 440–445.

Russell, S. and Gilson, L. (1995) *User Fees at Government Health Services: Is Equity Being Considered?* Public Health and Policy, London School of Hygiene and Tropical Medicine, London.

Save the Children Fund (1993) *Investing in Health – World Development Report 1993 : The SCF Perspective.* Save the Children Fund, London.

Tahzib, F. (1990) Nigeria: Talking about mothers. *Lancet,* **336**(8718): 802.

Van der Heijden, T. (1992) Letter. *Lancet,* **340**: 732.

WHO (1991) *Essential Elements of Obstetric Care at First Referral Level.* World Health Organization, Geneva.

WHO (1994) *Mother–Baby Package.* World Health Organization, Geneva.

World Bank (1993) *World Development Report 1993, Investing in Health.* Oxford University Press, New York.

Yoder, R.A. (1989) Are people willing and able to pay for health services? *Social Science and Medicine,* **29**(1): 35–42.

CHAPTER

5

Reducing Maternal Mortality from Abortion: The Midwife's Role in Abortion Care

Charlotte E. Hord and **Grace E. Delano**

INTRODUCTION

Induced abortion is one of the world's most common surgical procedures, with an estimated 36–53 million abortions performed annually (Henshaw and Morrow, 1990). There is very little risk involved when the procedure is performed by a trained and skilled provider under sanitary conditions; less risk, in fact, than is associated with childbirth (Gold, 1990). The death rate for first-trimester abortions in industrialized countries is now 0.6/100,000 procedures, making it safer than an injection of penicillin (Gold, 1990; Potts, 1993). In developing countries, however, the risk of death following unsafe abortion may be between 100 and 500 times higher than when the procedure is performed professionally under safe conditions (Wolf, 1994). The World Health Organization (WHO) offers a conservative estimate of 75,000 maternal deaths caused by unsafe abortion each year, though estimates are dramatically higher (WHO, 1994). Although these figures are staggering enough, they are based on hospital data and may reflect only a fraction of the total number of abortion-related deaths that occur in places with poor access to health care.

In this chapter the factors that contribute to high levels of maternal mortality from unsafe abortion are reviewed and the ways in which midwives can contribute to reducing maternal mortality by expanding their roles in the provision of abortion care are highlighted, with examples from different countries.

UNSAFE ABORTION

Despite the safety and simplicity of the abortion procedure, restrictive laws, policies, and practices limit access to safe abortion services for a majority of the world's women, even in countries that may have legal indications for abortion. When denied access to safe appropriate care, many women turn to unskilled providers to terminate unwanted pregnancies and often suffer complications that require medical intervention. Between 10 and 50% of all women who have an unsafe abortion need subsequent medical attention (WHO, 1994). The tragedy of this situation is compounded by limited opportunities for health-care professionals to obtain abortion-related training, leaving them unprepared to manage abortion complications safely. Given this multitude of obstacles, it is not surprising that unsafe abortion is the cause of 30–50% of all maternal deaths in Africa and Latin America (Odlind, 1993; Logie and Logie, 1994).

While maternal death may be the most drastic result of an unsafe abortion, it is far from the only negative consequence. For every woman who dies from an unsafe abortion, an estimated 10–15 experience related chronic pain or disability (Odlind, 1993) while 100 more suffer acute morbidity (Koblinsky *et al.*, 1992). Complications of abortion can develop into chronic pelvic inflammation, with associated permanent or recurrent pain, and/or secondary infertility due to tubal occlusion (Wolf, 1994). Severe damage to the uterus can necessitate a hysterectomy.

Unsafe abortion has a negative impact on health systems as well as on women's lives. The human and material costs of treating abortion complications can severely strain a health system's meagre resources, since complications almost always require uterine evacuation, and often necessitate blood transfusions, pain medication, antibiotics or other pharmaceuticals, and an overnight stay in hospital.

WHO HAS ABORTIONS?

Wherever there are men and women, there will be pregnancy and wherever there is pregnancy, there will be abortion.
Dr Khama Rogo, XIII FIGO World Congress, 1991

Women of all ages and social situations resort to abortion to regulate their fertility, usually as a solution to unwanted pregnancy; half of all pregnancies in the developing world are unwanted (Wolf, 1994). While in most industrialized countries abortion rates tend to be highest among single women aged 20–24, in parts of Africa women seeking abortion are frequently older and are seeking to delay or limit additional births (Jacobson, 1990; WHO, 1990). A 1987 study in Nigeria found that 34.8% of women who underwent an abortion were married, and 52.2% had two or more children (IPPF, 1994). Unwanted pregnancy may occur because a woman or her partner lack the knowledge of how to prevent or plan pregnancy, or because they lack access to effective, affordable, and acceptable contraceptives. 'Unwantedness' may be the result of cultural, religious, or even economic factors.

Abortion is exceedingly common, even when legal or cultural restrictions limit the availability of safe procedures. WHO estimates that approximately one induced abortion takes place for every three births; also, two of every five abortions are unsafe (Wolf, 1994). In Latin America, where elective abortion is largely prohibited by law, there are an estimated 3–7 million abortions induced annually, of which 85% are unsafe (Wolf, 1994). In Romania, where abortion and contraception were legalized in 1989, there were three times as many abortions as births in 1990 and 1991, primarily due to a lack of modern contraceptives, fears of their side-effects, and a history of reliance on abortion to regulate fertility (Hord *et al.*, 1991; Johnson *et al.*, 1993b).

As early sexual activity becomes more common in many parts of the world, adolescent numbers are increasing in abortion statistics. The mean age of first coitus in Africa is 13.5 years in boys and 14.5 years in girls. Of all African teenage girls, 75% become pregnant, 40% before the age of 17 (Logie and Logie, 1994). Many of these pregnancies result in abortion. In Nigeria, where abortion is legally permitted only to save the woman's life, a survey found that 30% of female secondary school students had undergone an abortion (IPPF, 1993). Similarly, a survey in Sierra Leone found that 44% of induced abortions were performed on teenage girls (CMA, 1993). Sadly, many of these abortions are performed both illegally and unsafely. Data from 13 African countries show that girls aged 11–19 account for 39–72% of all hospital admissions for abortion-related complications (IPPF, 1993).

WHY SHOULD THE MIDWIFE BECOME INVOLVED IN ABORTION CARE?

Midwives are health-care professionals dedicated to helping women maintain healthy reproductive lives. As the traditional role of the midwife is to give necessary supervision, care, and advice to women during pregnancy, labour, and the postpartum period (Kwast and Bentley, 1991), it is logical for women who experience complications related to pregnancy, including abortion, to seek care first from their local midwife. Most midwives, particularly those in private practice, already offer a variety of services that go beyond immediate pregnancy care. These range from basic preventive child health, such as immunizations and oral rehydration therapy, to provision of family planning and treatment of illness (GRMA, 1990). Midwives also fill an important information gap by educating the community about reproductive health issues, including how to safely regulate fertility and avoid unsafe abortion.

Unfortunately, despite their vital role in helping women maintain healthy reproductive lives, midwives are often prohibited from providing care for emergency life-threatening obstetric complications that are the major causes of maternal mortality, including abortion. Despite experiences that demonstrate midwives' ability to manage obstetric complications safely (Bhatia et al., 1980; Starrs, 1987; White et al., 1987), very few programmes provide training for or authorize midwives to manage these situations, forcing women to seek care from physicians or other providers that may be less accessible. A summary of safe motherhood strategies adopted by countries throughout the world consistently mentions unsafe abortion as a major contributor to maternal death and illness, but only a few countries have targeted training for midwives in abortion care as an appropriate intervention for addressing this problem directly (Otsea, 1992). This type of inaction, perhaps due to fear that such programmes would generate negative political and cultural reactions, means that women are allowed to die for lack of appropriate care.

WHY IS ABORTION CARE DIFFICULT TO FIND?

The concentration of health care in urban areas is one of the primary obstacles to women's access to timely and appropriate reproductive health services (Thaddeus and Maine, 1990). In the mountainous areas of Bali, Indonesia, where transport and access to primary or secondary health facilities are extremely limited, the maternal mortality rate is four times higher than in more centrally located areas (Potts, 1993).

In many developing countries, up to 80% of the population live in rural areas with limited access to health care (Kwast, 1991b). The distance women have to travel to seek reproductive health care, including abortion care, is an important factor in whether or not they will experience significant and long-term complications from an unsafe abortion.

Failing to train and adequately equip health-care staff to manage obstetric emergencies at the local level necessitates the referral of patients to already seriously overburdened centralized tertiary-care hospitals in urban areas, and forces patients who may be very ill to travel long distances in search of care.

Women may also have difficulty finding safe abortion care because health systems continue to rely on outdated procedures and unnecessarily restrictive service-delivery protocols. Treatment protocols for incomplete abortion throughout the developing world continue to endorse uterine evacuation by sharp curettage, also called dilatation and curettage or D&C, under heavy sedation or general anaesthesia. Since sharp curettage is usually performed in an operating theatre with general anaesthetic, which itself carries an additional risk of complications, treatment for incomplete abortion is often available only in tertiary or well-equipped secondary level hospitals. Many women suffering from incomplete abortion are in need of immediate life-saving care and may not survive the journey to a central hospital.

WHAT CAN BE DONE?

If you want to have an impact on reducing maternal mortality and you are committed to Safe Motherhood objectives, abortion is the single most important area to work in because it is preventable and you can make a difference.
Dr Khama Rogo, 1994 IPAS Africa Regional Trainers Meeting

A number of international professional organizations and bilateral donor agencies have begun to recognize the importance of the midwife's role in women's health and have endorsed midwives' greater involvement in a broader range of health services, including abortion care (Starrs, 1987; WHO, 1987; WHO, 1991b). The World Bank has advocated a three-point programme of pregnancy-related care that includes provision of safe abortion and other obstetric care by trained midwives (World Bank, 1993). Within this framework, staff should be trained to provide a "minimum package of essential clinical services," including antenatal and delivery care, and family planning. Although experienced physicians would have to supervise essential clinical care and to handle more complicated cases, the World Bank suggests that most services in the minimum package can be delivered by a nurse and/or midwife (World Bank, 1993). Similarly, recommendations of several international meetings, including the WHO Task Force on Human Resource Development for Maternal Health and Safe Motherhood and the Workshop on Midwifery Education that preceded the 1990 Triennial Congress of the International Confederation of Midwives (ICM), reflect the need for midwives to be trained in emergency uterine evacuation, a life-saving skills procedure (Kwast and Bentley, 1991; WHO, 1991b).

The 1991 Workshop on Obstetric and Maternity Care, a meeting convened in conjunction with the 1991 FIGO (International Federation of Gynaecology and Obstetrics) conference, also offered recommendations for empowering midwives to provide more comprehensive reproductive health care, including (Rooth and Kessel, 1992):

> *To prevent and manage the complications of abortion, available and acceptable contraception and referral for safe termination of an unwanted pregnancy [must be available at the primary health care level].*

MIDWIFERY EDUCATION

Why has it taken so long for the health-care community to recognize that midwives are skilled professionals capable of managing more than basic health care? One theory is that the policy of focusing medical education in teaching hospitals has restricted severely midwives' practice (Kwast, 1991b; Kwast and Bentley, 1991). Midwives who are supervised by physicians during practical training and taught to perform only standard, non-complicated procedures may have difficulty in practising with confidence when they are posted to a facility with no physician supervisor (Kwast, 1991b). Regardless of where it takes place, training that encourages a midwife to refer all complicated problems to a specialist, rather than teaching her to manage them herself, is not appropriate in countries with high maternal mortality where trained specialists are seldom available (Bentley, 1991).

The end result of this trend in hospital-based training is that midwives lack an awareness of the magnitude of maternal mortality and are not prepared to manage obstetric emergencies (Kwast, 1991b). Kwast calls for midwives to be trained urgently in the clinical skills necessary to manage essential obstetric functions, as defined by WHO (1991a), and in the prevention and management of the five major causes of maternal mortality: haemorrhage, obstructed labour, infection, toxaemia, and unsafe abortion. She argues that the skills reflected in *Essential Elements of Obstetric Care at First Referral Level* (WHO, 1991a) are no more esoteric or complex than other clinical skills and that an experienced midwife should be capable of learning and performing them with training (Murray, 1993). Margaret Marshall, Director of the Special Projects Section of the American College of Nurse-Midwives, appeals to policymakers to overturn laws that limit midwives' authority to practise emergency obstetric care. She argues that training for midwives must integrate traditional maternal and child health (MCH) and/or family planning (FP) services with skill-building in the management of obstetric complications, including treatment of sepsis and incomplete abortion, in order to enable midwives to treat women in a manner that will allow them to maintain healthy reproductive lives (Marshall, 1994a).

PROGRAMMATIC SOLUTIONS

Maine (1991) has proposed that any intervention designed to reduce maternal death and ill health must have an impact on at least one of three areas – preventing pregnancy, preventing the incidence of complications, and managing complications when they arise – all of which are factors in unsafe abortion. Midwives can have an impact on all three of these areas and, by so doing, can make a significant contribution to reducing maternal mortality. The following are suggestions for how midwives might become involved in abortion care:

- Midwives can learn to recognize the warning signs of incomplete abortion, provide emergency stabilization and resuscitation, and offer appropriate and timely referral for uterine evacuation.
- Midwives can learn to perform vacuum aspiration to treat incomplete abortion or to perform early induced abortion to decentralize care and reduce the need for referral to tertiary care settings.
- Midwives can provide family planning counselling and services, particularly to adolescents and to women who have experienced abortion and may be at high risk for future unintended pregnancies, but are not otherwise reached by family planning programmes.
- Midwives can work in under-served areas and make reproductive health services more available at low cost to rural women who currently lack access to care.
- Midwives can be educators and advocates for safer abortion care, including health education for women and families in their communities, and can work for policies and protocols that support the availability and accessibility of and need for safer abortion care.

The following sections describe regional and country-specific programmes and projects that address these five areas of action.

Stabilization and referral

Considering the grave problem that most rural women experience in having access to life-saving [care], the management of obstetric first aid should be the responsibility of all trained midwives.
Barbara Kwast (1990)

As they may be the first point of entry into the health system for women needing acute abortion care, it is vitally important that midwives learn to recognize the warning signs of incomplete abortion and to stabilize the woman's condition before referring her to another facility for uterine evacuation. Elements of stabilization and emergency resuscitation in the case of incomplete abortion include management of the airway and respiration, control of bleeding, intravenous fluid replacement, and control of pain (WHO, 1995).

An example of a programme designed to prepare midwives in emergency procedures is the Life-Saving Skills programme for midwives, developed by the American College of Nurse-Midwives and conducted in parts of Africa and Asia. Although much of the programme's curriculum is geared towards management of obstetric complications, such as the manual removal of the placenta and vacuum extraction, midwives are also taught life-saving techniques, such as resuscitation and fluid therapy. This programme has been remarkably successful in enhancing the ability of rural midwives and midwifery tutors to save the lives of women and infants (Marshall, 1994b).

BANGLADESH

Even when abortion is not the specific focus of an intervention, abortion-related mortality can decrease when midwives are prepared to manage complications promptly (Otsea, 1992). An example is a programme in Bangladesh which was designed to ensure that women with pregnancy-related complications receive appropriate and immediate stabilization and referral. The programme was generated in response to a study that identified unsafe abortion and other obstetric problems as the primary causes of death. Midwives in one area were trained in a variety of interventions, including administration of anti-eclamptic drugs, infusion of plasma-expanders in cases of haemorrhagic shock, and administration of antibiotics, and were assisted with transport when patients needed referral. Three years after the programme was implemented the maternal mortality ratio in the district had fallen by 68%. The cause of death that was reduced most dramatically by the programme was unsafe abortion (Otsea, 1992).

TURKEY

Midwives can also play an important role in ensuring access to abortion care in settings where abortion is legal by being aware of the indications for legal abortion and knowing where to refer women for these services. The Turkish abortion law was amended in 1983 to make abortion legal on request through the first 9 weeks of pregnancy. Although only obstetric and gynaecology (ob-gyn) specialists and certain general practitioners are allowed to perform the procedure, the Ministry of Health (MOH) recognized the important role that midwives can play in counselling and referral for services. Despite the liberal law, many women are unaware that early abortion services are available and wait until after the 9-week limit to seek care. In response to this problem the MOH has conducted special seminars for trainers at national nursing and midwifery schools, designed to provide student nurses and midwives with abortion-related skills early in their professional careers. The courses emphasize skills in abortion counselling, provide guidelines for when and where to refer women for services, and include basic clinical information about family planning counselling and methods (McLaurin *et al.*, 1991).

Performing uterine evacuation

We need to use appropriate technologies at all levels so that women have better care at lower costs.
Dr Fred Sai, Safe Motherhood Conference, 1987

Training and authorizing non-physician practitioners in supervised settings to perform uterine evacuation will reduce the need for long-distance travel by bringing abortion care closer to women; it may be an effective way to reach the women at highest risk of maternal mortality and morbidity (White *et al.*, 1987; Thaddeus and Maine, 1990). Midwives should be skilled in uterine evacuation and be able to manage emergency abortion complications and offer safe early induced abortion services. The most appropriate technology for low-resource settings, such as those in the developing world, is manual vacuum aspiration (MVA).

Numerous studies conducted over the past 20 years have shown that vacuum aspiration is the safest surgical technique for uterine evacuation in the first trimester (Greenslade *et al.*, 1993). In addition, vacuum aspiration is easier and faster to perform than sharp curettage, has half the complication rate (Grimes *et al.*, 1977; Greenslade *et al.*, 1993), and requires fewer hospital resources (Johnson *et al.*, 1992,

1993a; Blumenthal and Remsburg, 1994). WHO (1991a) includes vacuum aspiration as an essential element of care at the first-referral level.

MVA is a modified version of traditional electric vacuum aspiration, differing only in that the source of the vacuum is a hand-held syringe rather than an electric pump. MVA has been shown to improve the quality of care for patients treated for abortion (Bradley *et al.*, 1991) and is currently the procedure of choice for uterine evacuation among health-care providers in numerous countries throughout the world (BAPSA, 1985b; Kizza and Rogo, 1990; Ojo and Phido, 1991; Tolbert *et al.*, 1992; Ojo *et al.*, 1993). The simplicity of MVA enables it to be used safely and effectively by both trained physicians and non-physicians under the supervision of a physician (US Food and Drug Administration labelling for MVA instruments authorizes their use by or under the supervision of a physician). Authorizing supervised non-physician practitioners to perform uterine evacuation can increase women's access to treatment services and conserve resources without jeopardizing the quality of care offered (Greenslade *et al.*, 1993).

The following examples highlight the importance of the technology used to treat incomplete abortion and the benefits gained by changing clinical practice from sharp curettage to vacuum aspiration.

NIGERIA

In Nigeria, several university teaching hospitals began offering instruction in the use of MVA in 1987. When demand for MVA spread, two hospitals were designated as national training centres and began offering 1-week courses in the use of MVA and other aspects of high-quality abortion care. Statistics summarized after several years of MVA use at one of these training centres demonstrated the benefits that out-patient abortion case-management with MVA can bring to patients, providers, and the hospital (Shittu *et al.*, 1995).

Since 1987 a wide variety of health-care professionals have participated in the MVA programme in Nigeria, including nurses from government hospitals, private-sector midwives who run maternity homes, ob-gyn specialists and residents-in-training, and public- and private-sector general practitioners. The government of Nigeria supports MVA service delivery and considers it to be an important safe motherhood strategy. Currently, the Federal Ministry of Health is providing financial support to purchase MVA instruments and to provide MVA training to staff at secondary and tertiary hospitals in 22 states. In an effort to decentralize care even further, the Ministries of Health in eight states are now designing training and service delivery programmes to ensure that staff at secondary and first-referral hospitals can offer the appropriate abortion care.

BANGLADESH

Bangladesh has a long history of training non-physicians to use MVA to bring on delayed menses. Although induced abortion in Bangladesh is legally permitted only when pregnancy endangers the woman's life (BAPSA, 1985a), an estimated 750,000 women seek abortions each year, mostly clandestinely. At least 7500 die of complications, while several thousand become infertile or seriously ill (Otsea, 1992). To reduce the number of women seeking services from untrained or illegal providers, female community-based paramedical staff, called Family Welfare Visitors (FWV), are trained to provide family planning services and to perform MVA for legal menstrual regulation (MR) within a few weeks of a missed menstrual period. The FWVs must have completed 10 years of schooling, but usually have no prior medical experience. They undergo an 18-month family planning and maternal child health course, after which MR instruction is presented in an additional 3-week period (Dixon-Mueller, 1988). MR services in Bangladesh are estimated to save between 100,000 and 160,000 women from the dangers of unsafe abortion each year (Otsea, 1992). A 1980 study demonstrated that FWVs perform MVA safely with complication rates comparable to those of physicians (Bhatia *et al.*, 1980). Trained midwives, who are likely to have much greater familiarity than the average FWV with pregnancy and general reproductive health, can certainly provide these services at least as safely.

Family planning service delivery

The International Confederation of Midwives believes that every woman throughout her reproductive life should have accurate up-to-date information about, and access to, family planning. Inherent in this belief is the woman's right to choose. The midwife, by virtue of her education, her sphere of practice, and her unique relationship with women and their families, is in an ideal position to provide comprehensive family planning services.
ICM (1990), Statement on Planned Parenthood

Practising family planning is an effective means of avoiding many fertility-related health risks (World Bank, 1993); significant increases in contraceptive prevalence worldwide could result in notable reductions in the number of maternal deaths (Maine *et al.*, 1986; Herz and Measham, 1987). Midwives can play a major role in making family planning services more widely available. Because of their understanding of reproductive health needs and their unique relationship with women and their families, they are in an ideal position to provide women with comprehensive family planning care and information about reproductive health services, including abortion. Studies have shown that many women prefer to practise family planning than to use abortion to control their fertility (Johnson *et al.*, 1993b, 1995; Mutambirwa, 1994). Yet midwives, who are often the woman's first and main contact with the health system, are not providing these services as frequently as one might expect.

Community-based midwives are particularly important in the expansion of family planning services. Rural or low-income women may be the least likely to have access to a formal government-sponsored family planning facility, and may have no access to a family planning field worker who could provide information and simple services. In rural Uganda, for example, the travel time to the nearest family planning facility averages 1 hour, while in Guatemala 86% of rural women live in communities without family planning field staff (World Bank, 1993). Were rural midwives to offer family planning services, access to this important care could be greatly improved.

Adolescent fertility increasingly contributes to overall fertility. Pregnancies among adolescents often occur before marriage and are frequently unwanted. Interviews with teenage girls in Liberia, Mali, and Uganda in the 1980s showed that more than one in five had given birth to at least one child or was pregnant at the time of the interview (World Bank, 1993). Similarly, 16% of all births in 1992 in Latin America and Caribbean countries were to teenage girls (World Bank, 1993). In Ghana and Kenya, 40% of married teenagers who have children said their first pregnancy was unintended, while among unmarried teenagers in these countries the percentage of unintended births was 58% and 77%, respectively (World Bank, 1993). Family planning policies often discriminate against young or unmarried women, who may be the least informed about how to regulate their fertility safely. Midwives who offer family planning services should make a special effort to reach the adolescents in their community with counselling and advice about how to safely delay or plan child-bearing.

The following country examples reflect how midwives can contribute to improving maternal health through the provision of family planning counselling and services.

CHILE

Since the early 1960s, when the government of Chile officially included family planning in its maternal health programme, midwives have been authorized to provide contraceptive methods in addition to family planning information and counselling. This programme has resulted in dramatic improvements in the health of women and their families. Between 1960 and 1985 (Viel and Campos, 1987):

- Use of an effective modern contraceptive method by women of reproductive age increased from 1.2% to 24%.
- Infant mortality decreased from 120.3/1000 to 19.7/1000 live births.
- The number of women hospitalized for incomplete abortion per 1000 women of reproductive age fell from 29.8 to 11.
- Maternal mortality attributable to unsafe abortion fell from 35.7% to 24.7%.

GHANA

In 1987 the Ghana Registered Midwives Association (GRMA) embarked on a programme to train private midwives in family planning counselling, service delivery, and management, and to encourage them to incorporate these services into their maternity practices. While virtually all (98.5%) of the 134 midwives surveyed offered antenatal and delivery services at the time the programme began, only 11.4% also offered family planning. During the first 2 years of the programme, participating midwives collected 4462 data forms from clients to determine their needs and attitudes regarding family planning. Of these clients, 79.6% were using family planning for the first time, indicating that the midwives participating in this programme were providing services to a group that had not previously been reached. It was clear from the study that women and men from varying backgrounds wanted and were ready to accept family planning from private midwives (GRMA, 1990), whose services were easily accessible and whose fees were usually affordable.

Although offering family planning services may entail additional responsibilities and workload, the benefits that accrue to a private midwife are often significant and may outweigh any perceived negative aspects. The study in Ghana revealed, through in-depth follow-up interviews with the midwives who participated in the programme, that both their standing in the community and relationships with their clients improved when they began to offer family planning (GRMA, 1990).

Move to rural areas

Few rural health services have competent midwives assigned to them. Those that are so assigned, whilst competent as practitioners of normal midwifery, have often neither the skills nor the knowledge to deal with maternal health crises.
Barbara Kwast, 1990 ICM/WHO/UNICEF Pre-Congress Workshop on Midwifery Education

There is a severe shortage of trained midwives throughout the world (Kwast, 1991a, 1991b; Kwast and Bentley, 1991). Of 23 countries in Africa for which there are data, only seven are adequately staffed with midwives, while 16 need 21,000 more midwives (Kwast, 1991a, 1991b). The ratio of midwives to population, ranging from 1:30,000 to 1:300,000 in Africa and Asia, is far below the ideal of 1:5000 (Kwast and Bentley, 1991; Murray, 1993), and midwives are particularly scarce in rural areas (Murray, 1993).

Midwives could significantly improve the health of a majority of the world's women if they were equipped adequately to practise in community-based settings, as up to 80% of the population of most developing countries lives in rural areas (Kwast, 1991b). While midwives continue to work mostly in urban hospitals, offering services that could be delegated to other health workers, there are insufficient midwives in rural areas to provide adequate village services or to supervise the work of traditional birth attendants (Kwast, 1991b). Women seeking abortion care at their local health facility are unlikely to find personnel who have the skills to manage their problem, and may have to travel a great distance to find care.

Expanding services provided by midwives and other non-physicians is the only way to provide any health care to women and children in many rural villages. It is short-sighted to continue to deny these critical providers the training they need: midwives who staff rural health facilities must be trained and equipped to provide abortion care.

Advocacy and education

National midwifery associations should provide or advocate the provision of continuing education, whereby midwives can be trained to carry out life-saving functions. Midwives must take advantage of such training whether or not there is immediate financial gain.
Betts (1990), National Safe Motherhood Conference, Abuja, Nigeria

Despite a tendency to overlook or ignore unsafe abortion as a primary cause of maternal mortality, individuals who have been willing to speak out have succeeded in bringing this issue into discussions of safe motherhood. Regretfully, over the past few years very few of these voices have been those of midwives, perhaps because management of abortion is not typically considered to be one of a midwife's responsibilities. It is indisputable, however, that midwives do encounter women with problem pregnancies and are likely to need the skills to manage abortion complications at some point in their careers. The midwifery profession must begin to acknowledge the magnitude of the problem of unsafe abortion and to encourage a greater awareness among midwives of how they can work to reduce it (Odlind, 1993).

Midwives can contribute to this issue, both individually and as part of a larger group of professionals, by becoming advocates for policies and practices that encourage their role in safe and appropriate management for abortion-related problems. The individual midwife may have the most insight into the approaches to this problem that would be successful within her own local setting, and so she should identify ways in which she personally can work to improve abortion care. Collectively, midwives can contribute substantially by participating in professional associations. A recent regional meeting of the Commonwealth Medical Association (CMA) called for all health professionals, particularly nurses and doctors, to use their positions to advocate improvements in reproductive health and safe motherhood in their communities (CMA, 1993). Sadly, most governments fail to consult national professional health associations on health matters, or they consult physicians only, with the result that policies are set without the guidance of the complete health team, which includes midwives. Midwives who belong to professional associations must participate more actively and use their skills to organize and advocate for a greater voice in the health-care policies of their nations.

Midwives can also contribute by seeking opportunities to participate in local or national working groups on safe motherhood. Although unsafe abortion is frequently identified by these groups as a primary cause of maternal death and ill health, interventions designed by the groups rarely address the need to improve abortion care, and almost never involve midwives in the solution (Otsea, 1992). Midwives can be instrumental in lobbying for interventions that make use of the midwife.

If there is no vocal group or individual willing to advocate the need for midwives to become involved in abortion care, this area is likely to continue to be excluded from most midwifery training programmes and clinical protocols. In countries where midwifery training programmes are beginning to revise curricula to include a broader reproductive health focus or where patient management protocols are being established or adapted to reflect a focus on safe motherhood, midwives must make a case for the authority to manage obstetric emergencies without a physician present.

There is precedent for calling for these changes. Recent international conferences have highlighted the need to expand the midwife's educational opportunities and authority to practise in order to improve women's access to health care (WHO, 1991b, 1993). At an ICM Council meeting (May 1993), 19 member associations reported the need for revised curricula and advocated that a clinical component be maintained in midwifery education (ICM, 1994). Recommendations from the 1993 ICM/WHO/UNICEF workshop on 'Midwifery Practice – Measuring, Developing, and Mobilizing Quality of Care' included the following statement (WHO 1993):

> *[Countries must revise or enact legislation] that recognizes the scope of independent midwifery practice [so] the midwife is not constrained by others in her ability to evaluate and improve her practice. [Countries must] review and revise policies and job descriptions that govern the practice of midwifery to enable midwives to perform roles effectively in the promotion of safe motherhood.*

Finally, midwives must educate their clients about the dangers of unsafe abortion and ways to prevent unwanted pregnancy. As key providers of women's reproductive health care, midwives have a responsibility to provide accurate and complete information regarding all aspects of reproductive health, including abortion-related issues. In addition to providing basic information about prevention, midwives should ensure that women know which abortion care services exist and where they can be obtained, and believe in their effectiveness (Otsea, 1992).

CONCLUSION

According to WHO's Safe Motherhood Programme, during the late 1980s there was little or no improvement in coverage of maternity care or mortality from unsafe abortion (AbouZahr and Royston, 1992). Indeed, of 24 African countries surveyed recently, only two have managed to improve maternal mortality (Logie and Logie, 1994). It has been proposed that improving the availability of family planning, safe abortion, and emergency obstetric care is essential to ensure that maternal mortality decreases (Otsea, 1992). The midwife can contribute significantly to each of these areas.

The ICM and its colleague organizations have already strongly recommended broadening midwives' education and clinical skills, and expanding their responsibilities with respect to women's reproductive health care (WHO, 1987, 1991b; Rooth and Kessel, 1992). The approaches discussed here are but a few of the ways midwives can address the problem of unsafe abortion and improve maternal health. These goals are achievable.

Midwives can be instrumental in implementing specific interventions that can reduce both the reliance on and the negative impact of unsafe abortion. In situations where midwives are not permitted to manage cases of incomplete abortion and offer uterine evacuation services, they can perform a valuable service by recognizing the condition and stabilizing the patient before referring her to another facility for treatment. When midwives are trained and authorized to perform uterine evacuation, they can offer safe induced abortion services where legal, or can manage incomplete abortion promptly, rather than referring women to tertiary care centres for treatment. Midwives are in the position to offer family planning counselling and services to all their female clients, particularly to adolescents and to those who have experienced an abortion. Midwives must provide care in the communities where they are needed most. Finally, midwives must become more vocal about the need for more appropriate regulations regarding who can provide abortion care, and must work to promote the availability of more accessible and decentralized services.

The ICM and other professional institutions have promoted policies that authorize midwives to provide life-saving services, including safe and appropriate abortion care. When national policymakers and local midwives' organizations follow this example and policies and practices begin to reflect such recommendations, midwives will be better prepared to contribute to breaking the cycle of unwanted pregnancy and repeat abortion and to reducing high maternal mortality rates among the women they serve.

ACKNOWLEDGEMENTS

The authors thank Merrill Wolf and Marian Abernathy of IPAS for commenting on early versions of this paper, and Veronica Williams for her invaluable bibliographic assistance.

REFERENCES

AbouZahr, C. and Royston, E. (1992) Excessive hazards of pregnancy and childbirth in the Third World. *World Health Forum,* **13**(4): 343–345.

BAPSA (1985a) *MR Newsletter,* Number 1, Bangladesh Association for Prevention of Septic Abortion, Dhaka.

BAPSA (1985b) *MR Newsletter,* Number 3, Bangladesh Association for Prevention of Septic Abortion, Dhaka.

Bentley, J. (1991) Teamwork is Essential. *World Health Forum,* **12**(1): 11–14.

Betts, G.A. (1990) *The Midwife's Role in the Control of Maternal Mortality.* Paper presented at Society of Obstetrics and Gynaecology of Nigeria (SOGON) Safe Motherhood Conference, Abuja, Nigeria.

Bhatia, S., Faruque, A.S.G., and Chakraborty, J. (1980) Assessing menstrual regulation performed by paramedics in rural Bangladesh. *Studies in Family Planning,* **11**(6): 213–218.

Blumenthal, P.D. and Remsburg, R.E. (1994) A time and cost analysis of the management of incomplete abortion with manual vacuum aspiration. *International Journal of Gynecology and Obstetrics,* **45**: 261–267.

Bradley, J., Sikazwe, N., and Healy, J. (1991) Improving abortion care in Zambia. *Studies in Family Planning,* **22**(6): 391–394.

CMA (1993) *Manual on Reproductive Health and Safe Motherhood.* Report of a Training Workshop for the West Africa Region, Commonwealth Medical Association, London.

Dixon-Mueller, R. (1988) Innovations in reproductive health care: Menstrual regulation policies and programs in Bangladesh. *Studies in Family Planning,* **19**(3): 129–140.

Gold, R. (1990) *Abortion and Women's Health: A Turning Point for America?* The Alan Guttmacher Institute, New York.

GRMA (1990) *Final Report: Operations Research Project,* Ghana Registered Midwives Association, Accra, Ghana.

Greenslade, F.C., Leonard, A.H., Benson, J., Winkler, J., and Henderson, V.L. (1993) *Manual Vacuum Aspiration: A Summary of Clinical and Programmatic Experience.* IPAS, Carrboro, NC.

Grimes, D.A., Schulz, K.F., Cates, W. Jr, and Tyler, C.W. Jr (1977) The Joint Program for the Study of Abortion/CDC: A Preliminary Report. In: Hern, W. and Andrikopoulos, B. (eds), *Abortion in the Seventies.* National Abortion Federation, New York.

Henshaw, S.K. and Morrow, E. (1990) *Induced Abortion: A World Review. 1990 Supplement.* The Alan Guttmacher Institute, New York.

Herz, B. and Measham, A.R. (1987) *The Safe Motherhood Initiative: Proposals for Action.* World Bank, Washington, DC.

Hord, C.E., David, H.P., Donnay, F., and Wolf, M. (1991) Reproductive health in Romania: Reversing the Ceausescu legacy. *Studies in Family Planning,* **22**(4): 231–240.

ICM (1990) *Planned Parenthood.* Ref: 90/5/PP, adopted by the International Confederation of Midwives Council, Kobe, October 1990.

ICM (1994) *ICM Newsletter,* **7**(1): 5. International Confederation of Midwives.

IPPF (1993) *1992–93 Annual Report.* International Planned Parenthood Federation, London.

IPPF (1994) *Unsafe Abortion and Post-Abortion Family Planning in Africa.* The Mauritius Conference, International Planned Parenthood Federation, London.

Jacobson, J.L. (1990) *The Global Politics of Abortion.* Worldwatch Paper 97, The Worldwatch Institute, Washington, DC.

Johnson, B.R., Benson, J., and Leibson Hawkins, B. (1992) Reducing resource use and improving quality of care with MVA. *Advances in Abortion Care,* **2**(2). IPAS, Carrboro, NC.

Johnson, B.R., Benson, J., Bradley, J., and Rábago Ordoño, A. (1993a) Costs and resource utilization for the treatment of incomplete abortion in Kenya and Mexico. *Social Science and Medicine*, **36**(11): 1443–1453.

Johnson, B.R., Horga, M., and Andronache, L. (1993b) Contraception and abortion in Romania. *Lancet*, **341**: 875–878.

Johnson, B.R., Horga, M., and Andronache, L. (1995) Women's perspectives on abortion in Romania. *Social Science and Medicine*, to be published.

Kizza, A.P.M. and Rogo, K.O. (1990) Assessment of the manual vacuum aspiration (MVA) equipment in the management of incomplete abortion. *East African Medical Journal*, **67**(11): 812–821.

Koblinsky, M.A., Timyan, J., and Gay, J. (eds) (1992) *The Health of Women: A Global Perspective.* Westview Press, Boulder.

Kwast, B.E. (1990) International Congress of the International Federation of Midwives, October 7–12, Kobe, Japan.

Kwast, B.E. (1991a) Midwives' role in safe motherhood. *Journal of Nurse-Midwifery*, **36**(6): 366–372.

Kwast, B.E. (1991b) Safe motherhood: A challenge to midwifery practice. *World Health Forum*, **12**(1): 1–6.

Kwast, B.E. and Bentley, J. (1991) Introducing confident midwives: Midwifery education – Action for safe motherhood. *Midwifery*, **7**: 8–19.

Logie, A.W. and Logie, D.E. (1994) Women's health in Africa. *Lancet*, **343**: 170.

Maine, D. (1991) *Safe Motherhood Programs: Options and Issues.* Columbia University Center for Population and Family Health, New York.

Maine, D., Rosenfield, A., Kimball, A.M., Kwast, B., Papiernik, E., and White, S. (1986) *Maternal Mortality in Developing Countries: Program Options and Practical Considerations.* Background paper prepared for the International Safe Motherhood Conference, Nairobi, Kenya, February 1987.

Marshall, M. (1994a) Pregnancy, labor, and delivery care: Life saving skills and family planning programs. In: *Reproductive Health Approach to Family Planning.* Presentations from a panel held on Professional Development Day at the USAID Cooperating Agency Meeting, Washington, DC, 1994, compiled by the Population Council, New York.

Marshall, M. (1994b) Personal communication.

McLaurin, K.E., Hord, C.E., and Wolf, M. (1991) Health systems' role in abortion care: the need for a pro-active approach. *Issues in Abortion Care 1.* IPAS, Carrboro, NC.

Murray, S.F. (1993) Appropriate training for midwives. *NU Nytt om U-Landshalsovard*, **7**: 33–36.

Mutambirwa, J. (1994) *Unwanted Pregnancy, Abortion and Post-Abortion Family Planning in Zimbabwe.* Final Report to IPAS, Carrboro, NC, unpublished.

Odlind, V. (1993) Induced abortion – A short overview of a worldwide maternal health problem. *NU Nytt om U-Landshalsovard*, **7**:15–17.

Ojo, O.A. and Phido, F. (1991) *Evaluation of Manual Vacuum Aspiration Training Programmes and Subsequent Clinical Use of the Procedure at Ahmadu Bello University Teaching Hospital and Lagos University Teaching Hospital, Nigeria.* Paper presented at 1991 Annual Conference of the Society of Obstetrics and Gynaecology of Nigeria (SOGON), Lagos, Nigeria, unpublished.

Ojo, O.A., Phido, F., Hord, C.E., Benson, J., and Wingate, I. (1994) *An Evaluation of Provider Acceptability and Use of Manual Vacuum Aspiration (MVA) in Nigeria.* Copies can be obtained from IPAS, Carrboro, NC.

Otsea, K. (1992) *Progress and Prospects. The Safe Motherhood Initiative 1987–1992.* Background document for The Meeting of Partners for Safe Motherhood, World Bank, Washington, DC.

Potts, M. (1993) Family planning, demography and safe motherhood. *NU Nytt om U-Landshalsovard,* **7**: 7–10.

Rooth, G. and Kessel, E. (eds) (1992) Workshop on obstetric and maternity care. *International Journal of Gynecology and Obstetrics,* **38**(Suppl.).

Shittu, S.O., Ifenne, D.I., and Ekwempu, C.C. (1995) Transformation of uterine evacuation in a Nigerian teaching hospital. *Nigerian Medical Journal,* in press.

Starrs, A. (1987) *Preventing the Tragedy of Maternal Deaths.* A Report on the International Safe Motherhood Conference, World Bank, Washington, DC.

Thaddeus, S. and Maine, D. (1990) *Too Far to Walk: Maternal Mortality in Context.* Columbia University, New York.

Tolbert, K., Chambers, V., and Saldaña, A. (1992) *Study of Sustainability and Quality of MVA Services in Zacatecas.* Presented at the Reunión de Evaluación del Programa de AMEU en el Estado de Zacatecas, Zacatecas, Mexico.

Viel, B. and Campos, W. (1987) La experiencia Chilena de mortalidad infantil y materna, 1940–1985. *Perspectivas Internacionales en Planificación Familiar,* Número Especial.

White, S.M., Thorpe, R.G., and Maine, D. (1987) Emergency obstetric surgery performed by nurses in Zaire. *Lancet,* **ii**(8559): 612–613.

WHO (1987) *Report of ICM/WHO/UNICEF Pre-Congress Workshop on Women's Health and the Midwife: A Global Perspective.* WHO/MCH/87.5, World Health Organization, Geneva.

WHO (1990) *Abortion: A Tabulation of Available Data on the Frequency and Mortality of Unsafe Abortion.* WHO/MCH/90.14, World Health Organization, Geneva.

WHO (1991a) *Essential Elements of Obstetric Care at First Referral Level.* World Health Organization, Geneva.

WHO (1991b) *Midwifery Education: Action for Safe Motherhood.* Report of a Collaborative Pre-Congress Workshop, Kobe, Japan, 5–6 October, 1990, WHO/MCH/91.3, World Health Organization, Geneva.

WHO (1993) *Safe Motherhood: A Newsletter of Worldwide Activity,* Issue 13. World Health Organization, Geneva.

WHO (1994) *Abortion: A Tabulation of Available Data on the Frequency and Mortality of Unsafe Abortion,* 2nd edn. WHO/FHE/MSM/93.13, World Health Organization, Geneva.

WHO (1995) *Complications of Abortion. Technical and Managerial Guidelines for Prevention and Treatment.* World Health Organization, Geneva.

Wolf, M. (1994) Consequences and prevention of unsafe abortion: Report of two panels at the XIII World Congress of Gynaecology and Obstetrics, Singapore, 1991. *Issues in Abortion Care 3,* IPAS, Carrboro, NC.

World Bank (1993) *World Development Report 1993.* Oxford University Press, Washington, DC.

Postpartum Family Planning Services: Challenges for the Future

Patricia Semeraro

Postpartum family planning programmes have historically suffered from a failure to take into account mothers' concerns and have lacked co-ordination with the child health services. In this chapter it is argued that there has been an inappropriate degree of emphasis on immediate contraceptive care before discharge from the maternity hospital, and a lack of imagination concerning appropriate alternatives. Midwives at provider, programme manager, and policymaker levels face a key challenge to develop those alternatives.

POSTPARTUM CARE – WHAT DOES IT MEAN?

While we have a fair idea of what 'family planning services' means, the meaning of specifically 'postpartum' contraceptive care is actually a lot less clear. In fact, the word 'postpartum' has a meaning so inexact that a fair amount of confusion has been caused. "Despite its Latin origin suggesting scientific precision, the term 'postpartum' has no specific definition with regard to the health care of mothers and babies immediately following childbirth" (Winikoff and Mensch, 1991). Postpartum as defined in Webster's *New Collegiate Dictionary* is "a period following parturition." This definition has a time dimension, but clearly lacks specificity. What time period is meant by postpartum? "The minutes, hours, days, or, in many cases, the first six weeks following a birth have all been called the postpartum period" (Winikoff and Mensch, 1991).

The word 'postpartum' has been used in many different ways. The term has been defined from an administrative focus as the length of stay in the hospital after delivery or the length of time in the delivery room after expulsion of the placenta. Others define the term physiologically – the time it takes for the uterus to involute to its pre-pregnancy shape and size. The term 'postpartum' has been defined by some cultures as the period from immediately after childbirth to when normal activities are resumed.

In Tunisia, the postpartum period is defined as a one of convalescence for 40 days after delivery; the fortieth day marks an end to this period of rest and the beginning of resumption of normal activities. With respect to timing, it has also been defined as the period during which particular health services are provided (for example, family planning services or post-birth check-ups for mothers.)

In addition, the concept of what constitutes the postpartum period is shaped by cultural systems. In many non-Western societies the postpartum period is often seen as a time for restoring the new mother to the life of the community. It is seen as a vulnerable time, and the emphasis is on the care of the mother. The woman is relieved of her ordinary tasks. Community involvement and support may be extensive. In contrast, in many Western societies these aspects have been lost. The postpartum period is simply seen as the period from delivery of the placenta to the 6-week check-up, with little connection to previous or subsequent events and care. Potential stresses on the mother are largely ignored, and there is often no community involvement or support.

'POSTPARTUM' FAMILY PLANNING STRATEGIES

Demographers have described various strategies for the timing of postpartum contraception (Potter *et al.*, 1973, 1979). The strategies are:

- A 'postpartum strategy', in which contraception is adopted immediately.
- A 'post-amenorrhoeal strategy', in which contraception is adopted after first menses.
- A 'fixed duration strategy', in which contraception is adopted a set number of months (T) after childbirth.
- A 'mixed T strategy', in which contraception is adopted T months after childbirth or after first menses, whichever occurs first.

Evaluations of postpartum family planning strategies must be interpreted in the light of fecundity and contraceptive characteristics (contraceptive discontinuation and length of amenorrhoea). The goal should be to adopt a service paradigm that is truly responsive to the desire of its potential clients. In the long run, the aims should be to increase the options available to women and to ensure flexibility of timing to enable the use of health services generally and for the adoption of contraception in particular.

THE HISTORY OF POSTPARTUM CONTRACEPTIVE CARE

A look back at the history of postpartum family planning programmes reveals that the concept is not a new one. The first organized postpartum programme was in 1930 at Johns Hopkins Hospital in Baltimore, Maryland (Zatuchni, 1970). Over the next 30 years, little attention was paid to the 'postpartum' women. In the mid 1960s, the Population Council began a demonstration project aimed at providing family planning services to women after childbirth or abortion. Acclaimed as a great success by family planning professionals, the programme became known as the 'International Postpartum Program'. Many more experimental programmes sprang up in over 21 countries (Taylor and Berelson, 1970; Castadot *et al.*, 1975). These experimental programmes demonstrated that such services are feasible, effective, and affordable in large urban hospitals and rural demonstration projects.

However, despite this success, the early postpartum programmes remained as demonstrations. Some of the early sites dropped out of the programme or reduced the accessibility of a range of postpartum family planning services. At the same time, the family planning field shifted its focus to the development of other delivery systems (i.e., out-patient family planning clinics, community-based distribution, and social marketing systems). By the 1980s, virtually all research specifically directed at postpartum programmes had disappeared from family planning literature. But now, in the 1990s, there appears to be a renewed enthusiasm for more explicit attention to immediate postpartum services, and it seems important that midwives reconsider the value of and their role in such services.

The assumptions behind postpartum family planning services

First, the prevailing assumption behind most postpartum family planning services has been that women are most receptive to contraceptive use immediately after the birth of a child. Childbirth is thought to have been an unpleasant experience, increasing a woman's motivation to avoid another pregnancy, labour, and delivery in the near future. Second, it has been assumed that women 'cannot be depended upon' to return for family planning services and, therefore, family planning must be offered soon after delivery.

There is little concrete evidence for the first assumption. In fact, very little systematic work has been done on the subject of maternal motivation. We are just beginning to see the results of research that address the issue of what women want and when they want it. Data from Turkey (Bulut and Molzan, 1993) suggest that family planning information *alone* does not satisfy the needs of the majority of women. Indeed, it appears that mothers often have immediate concerns that are far more pressing than avoiding another pregnancy. Focus groups and questionnaires were used to elicit data on women's needs and wants for services during the postpartum period. Overall, the most common answer was information on infant care. Also, substantial numbers of women wanted information on family planning and breastfeeding. Few desired information on their own health.

Women users and providers also seemed to have fairly different emphases with respect to services or the most appropriate time to adopt contraception. Providers thought 'immediately' was a good idea, but none of the women did; on the other hand, many women identified 'post-menstruation' as a good time to begin.

The second assumption, that women do not return for medical services after childbirth, is disputed by recent evidence. If programmes are well run and provide the desired services, women will return to use them (Coeytaux, 1989).

Problems also arise when programme administrators impose unnecessarily restrictive protocols, so that many women who would like family planning services cannot obtain them. Even when services do attempt to address mothers' concerns, rigid medical norms sometimes prevent women from obtaining a contraceptive method. Some of these norms are related to attempts to avoid providing contraceptives to women who are already pregnant. They ignore, however, a good deal of basic biological information about the risks of pregnancy in lactating women in the early postpartum period. These risks have been demonstrated to be extraordinarily low. A programme that insists a woman must resume menses before she can be given certain types of effective contraceptives is, in fact, increasing the risk of unplanned pregnancy among its clients.

A Postpartum Program (Coeytaux, 1989) was set up in the Maternal and Neonatal Hospital in Sfax, Tunisia, to improve the quality of post natal care. It was found that approximately half of the women left the clinic without being given a contraceptive method. One reason for this was gynaecological abnormalities (i.e., vaginal discharge and cervical inflammation). The protocol at the Sfax Maternity was to refer for treatment women with a suspected vaginal infection. They were given a prescription and instructed to return for a follow-up examination and the contraceptive method 2 weeks later. A second major reason for women leaving the clinic without a method was that they had not yet resumed their menses. Sfax medical protocol prohibits the insertion of an intrauterine device (IUD) or prescription of oral contraceptives until menses has resumed. This may have serious consequences for both mothers and their children if women are thwarted in their attempts to avoid a subsequent closely spaced birth.

Postpartum family planning programmes historically have suffered from a number of deficiencies:

- A failure by health professionals to learn about and take into account mothers' concerns in the design of postpartum services.
- A lack of knowledge among many health professionals about breastfeeding and, as a result, inadequate contraceptive advice and services for lactating women.
- A lack of co-ordination between child health and family planning services, resulting in a failure to design service packages that offer health care to mothers and children at the same time (well-child immunization, breastfeeding support, contraceptive services for mothers).

ELEMENTS OF SUCCESSFUL POSTPARTUM FAMILY PLANNING PROGRAMMES

Family Health International (FHI) at the International Conference on Postpartum Contraception held in Mexico City in 1990 proposed two important characteristics necessary for postpartum family planning programmes to be effective:

- Variety of contraceptive options.
- Integration of contraceptive services with other services that promote mother–infant health in general.

Program data from the Sfax postpartum programme in Tunisia suggest that the kinds of services offered, as well as sensitivity to the local cultural practices of the population, are the key to the success of any family planning programme. Coeytaux (1989) highlighted several aspects of the Sfax programme that have contributed to its success:

- Linkage of postpartum appointment day to a culturally significant date. In most Muslim cultures, a rest of 40 days after delivery is considered essential for the convalescence of the mother and the development of the infant. During this period, the mother is carefully protected. She does not leave her home and is relieved of all household responsibilities, except that of tending to her new-born infant. The fortieth day marks the end of this postpartum period of convalescence. Then, according to tradition, the mother may resume her household responsibilities and appear in public. Traditionally, a celebration is held on the fortieth day as well, marking the end of the mother's convalescence and the beginning of a normal routine for both mother and child. By linking the follow-up visit with this culturally significant day, the Sfax Centre managed to incorporate the postpartum visit into the day's observances. (As this timing is meaningful to the family, the date is easily remembered. Most women do return exactly 40 days after delivery; those whose fortieth day falls on a Sunday are told to return the following Monday.) Coincidentally, this day correlates well with the usual Western medical recommendation of a '6-week' postpartum visit.

- Appropriate timing of delivery of contraceptive services. In Tunisia, by the fortieth day following birth, women are ready to think about contraception; they have completed their postpartum recovery period and the infant is well established. They are not asked to adopt a contraceptive early in the postpartum period.
- Focus: *the mother–infant dyad.* This is perhaps the most important innovation of the Sfax programme. Since a mother with a new-born child has to take the child with her when she goes for medical services for herself, it is much more convenient to be able to obtain all health services at the same time and in the same place. The mother no longer has to wonder where to leave her baby, who will take care of the baby, or whether the baby is welcome at the clinic. This seemingly small detail was mentioned by many women as one of the attractions of the service. By keeping the infant beside her during her examination, the mother feels more secure and does not experience the anxiety many women feel when they do not know where their infants are and how they are faring.
- Commitment and motivation of staff and programme managers.

In his overview of the Senegalese Health Care System, Mohamadou Fall (1992) suggests that integration of maternal and infant health services is necessary to improve the overall quality of services. The Institut du Pediatrie Sociale (Institute of Paediatric Health) in Senegal is currently implementing a new strategy to integrate maternal and infant health services. As part of this integrated postpartum health care programme for mothers and their babies, the general health of mother and infant, child growth and development, mother's breast milk availability, nutritional status, immunizations, and family planning needs are all checked and documented during visits. Such an approach to service provision will, it is hoped, encourage continued contraceptive use and will make it easier for women to overcome cultural barriers to family planning, since family planning will be seen as part of a broader programme aimed at improving the overall health of mothers and their babies.

The effectiveness of another postpartum health care and family planning programme in Santiago, Chile (Diaz, 1992) is based on many factors, including:

- Mother and child are viewed as a unit. Mothers and their children have the same number of postpartum visits scheduled on the same days.
- Providers work together as a team.
- Education and counselling is a central component of the programme.
- A variety of contraceptive methods are offered with a special emphasis on those methods that do not interfere with lactation and infant growth.
- Breastfeeding promotion.

WOMEN'S CHANGING NEEDS

Only recently has data been collected on women's desires regarding timing and type of contraception. But as Mensch (1992) points out, women manifest various desires and behaviours in the postpartum period, so a variety of strategies are needed. A programme that promotes not only a choice of methods, but also a choice of timing may be the answer. A postpartum programme that provides contraceptive information at all times and family planning services at delivery and anytime thereafter may better address the needs of women. A programme that is based on the concepts of education and counselling, the mother–infant dyad, integration of breastfeeding into birth-spacing strategies and cultural awareness may better encompass the total picture of what women want.

GOALS AND OPPORTUNITIES FOR PROGRAMME DESIGN

Family planning services are shifting emphasis from a demographic orientation to a focus on the needs of clients. The aim of family planning programmes is to help as many couples as possible achieve their reproductive goals. The question that arises is which service paradigm produces the best outcome. The response depends on the setting and is determined by breastfeeding behaviour, duration of contraceptive use, ability to return to a service delivery point, and the types of services available. Whether a given system or approach to service is maximally functional depends on the circumstances and the context. If programmes are effective, the next question we need to ask is are they cost-effective. The cost-effectiveness of a postpartum programme is related to factors that can influence the satisfaction of users or the costs of services. Various factors can influence programme costs:

- Timing (for example, provision of a contraceptive method before hospital discharge or later in the postpartum period).
- Rate of return for postpartum visits or other follow-up visits (the less the number of visits the more cost-effective).
- Continuation rates of contraceptive methods (the higher the continuation rates of a method, the more cost-effective).
- Cost of the contraceptive provided.
- Constellation of postpartum services (the more services a client receives for a given cost the greater the cost benefit).
- Labour costs (for example, different labour costs for different levels of health care workers).

Major issues for postpartum programme design in the 1990s

Planners and service providers concerned about developing appropriate family planning provision for postpartum women need to take into account the following:

- *A focus on health systems rather than individual service sites.* Traditionally, postpartum programmes have functioned as demonstration projects within individual service sites. While this model is extremely useful in the introduction of the service strategy, it quickly becomes obsolete unless the programme is replicated at other hospitals. The issue of sustainability and the capacity of a programme to continue to provide valued services over time at a reasonable cost are critical in light of increasingly limited resources.

- *Systems should include private as well as public sources.* Traditionally, postpartum contraceptive services have been provided in public sector institutions, given their large client population; their access to public sector resources, facilities, and staff; and their capacity to institutionalize the programme from a financial as well as policy perspective (AVSC, 1989). The extension of the postpartum family planning model should include private as well as public services, particularly where public services are limited or of poor quality. World-wide, there has not been much movement from the public to the private sector during the past two decades. Sample surveys on sources of supply of contraceptive services and commodities indicate that 50–75% of users obtain their contraceptive supplies from public sources. By increasing the role of the private sector, we supplement the health infrastructure and give clients alternative sources of supplies. The ready availability of contraceptive methods attracts additional users; thus, in many settings alternative modes of distribution increase use. For example, a study conducted in Ghana estimated that private maternity clinics provided about as much prenatal care as did the region's entire government health system. However, few maternity clinics provided family planning services, largely because the midwife–proprietors had never been encouraged to do so. Following a training effort, 8479 users were recruited from 12,131 deliveries. Of these, 80% were first-time users, and the continuation rate among these users was 69% at 9 months' postpartum (CPFH, 1989). Recently, Indonesia instituted a programme to increase the role of the private sector. Early reports suggest this effort is succeeding.
- *The focus should be on rural as well as urban populations.* Here a number of questions have yet to be answered. Can postpartum programmes employed in urban hospital settings be adapted to home deliveries in rural areas? Can existing postpartum programmes facilitate the development of mechanisms for serving more rural populations? What role can midwives play?
- *Programmes should consider the adoption of a postpartum strategy based on the concept of 'method mix'.* This type of approach uses different methods to meet the different needs of women at different stages of the postpartum period. It would incorporate choice and respond to a woman's own sense of timing.
- *Systems should incorporate breastfeeding into postpartum family planning strategies.* In the past, we have often ignored the contraceptive effect of breastfeeding. Yet the lactational amenorrhoea method (LAM), which relies on exclusive and frequent breastfeeding, is more than 98% effective in protecting against a pregnancy if the woman is in the first 6 months postpartum and is still amenorrhoeic (Kennedy *et al.*, 1989). Adoption of amenorrhoea as an explicit family planning strategy is not generally accepted by health professionals. Sally Tom (1992) notes that non-acceptance of LAM may be due to its divergence from the usual medical model of contraception: no medical procedure or prescription is needed. The method is client-controlled and information-based. Recognizing LAM as an effective method, however, legitimizes a traditional and natural means of child spacing. Where there are problems with the acceptability of other methods, LAM may help close the gap between traditional beliefs and modern methods of child spacing. The important questions regarding its incorporation into postpartum services revolve around whether the service providers can learn about LAM and transmit this information

in an accurate and comprehensible way to women and whether women can then both understand and use this information (Winikoff and Mensch, 1991).

- *Planners should recognize the effects of modernization on postpartum health care.* Modernization has caused extreme fragmentation in service delivery systems. This has hindered the progress towards integration of maternal and infant health care services. Modernization has also brought changes in the ways we construct and understand the postpartum period, who controls it, and how disease and appropriate care are defined. It has brought changes (1) in the structure and strength of support networks to the expectant and new mother, shifting the burden for providing physical and emotional support from traditional kinship networks to the conjugal unit; (2) in concepts of time, with a shift to institutional time, which fits the needs of health care providers and employers better than it does the needs of new mothers; and (3) in the dominant mode of knowing, with empirical knowledge replacing spiritual knowledge (Rogow, 1992).

- *Providers must recognize the need to prevent sexually transmitted diseases (STDs) and human immunodeficiency virus (HIV) transmission.* With the rapid and worrisome rise in the transmission of the HIV virus, some family planning institutions have begun to incorporate information and education for both providers and clients about STDs and HIV/AIDS with family planning services. Infections of the reproductive tract, including the common STDs and HIV infection, are of central concern to the providers of family planning service, as these infections influence the safety and quality of service programmes and impact on the demand for fertility regulation and utilization of contraceptive methods (Elias, 1993). Also, the increased consciousness of STDs has highlighted the need to consider the capacities of contraceptive methods to protect against infection alongside their effectiveness in preventing pregnancy.

THE ROLE OF MIDWIVES

The midwife has a role in postpartum programmes at any of three levels – as a key provider of family planning services, as a programme manager, and as a policymaker. Midwives are in a special position to know what women want and can do much to clarify and illuminate women's perceptions of services in the postpartum period. As Winikoff (1992) has noted, a woman is only one person, but she must respond in an integrated way to the multiple demands of her body, her new child, her sexual relationship, and her partner. She must also respond to her obligations as provider and nurturer in a family and perhaps to other economic, social, and ceremonial obligations. It is the responsibility of midwives and other service providers to recognize this and to provide appropriate information and education – information that gives women a sense of control and promotes healthy behaviour. The midwife needs to assess each woman individually with regard to age, fertility status, number of children, health, coital patterns, religious beliefs, and local customs, and whether or not she intends to breastfeed fully. Then the woman, along with her provider, must attempt to match her specific needs and desires with the safest and most effective contraceptive available.

As programme managers, midwives must make every effort to provide avenues for dialogue and interchange among clients, health providers, and policymakers. Only through this exchange of ideas can we hope to provide a *total* reproductive health programme that includes the kind of services women truly want and need. As managers, midwives need to know what services can be combined with different health care systems and how systems operating currently provide health care for mothers and children after birth. They need to provide leadership and support to experimental postpartum services. But leadership and support are not enough in themselves. As Townsend and Tolbert (1990) have pointed out, programme directors need clearly stated operational policies. These policies serve to connect specific service activities with their organizational units and budgets. It is these policies that facilitate the in-service training programmes needed to prepare staff to work as members of the reproductive health care team. They serve to guide the process of integration and allow models for service delivery to develop and later be replicated.

As policymakers, midwives must be change agents. Obstacles to the general integration of women's health care services are many. Lack of knowledge and expertise on the part of the provider, logistics, cost, and, in some cases, cultural and political prejudice against family planning, are but a few of the obstacles to successful integration of various postpartum services.

Faundes (1992) encourages policymakers to take advantage of existing factors that favour integration. For example, current mother–child health staff can be cross-trained to provide a full scope of women's health services. Training should not only provide for technical-skill acquisition and dissemination of specific information, but should also cover health planning and social medicine. This training will communicate to the health providers the benefits of service integration. Components for increasing and maintaining the motivation of health providers to integrate postpartum health care services are important, and include on-going supervision and the interaction of providers with organized community groups. As policymakers, midwives should be involved in the research efforts that re-examine women's needs and desires in the postpartum period and the possibilities for expanded service delivery options.

The role of midwifery in postpartum family planning programmes in the next decade is as multidimensional as the kind of services we hope to provide.

ACKNOWLEDGEMENT
Much of the material for the first two sections is drawn from Winikoff and Mensch (1991).

REFERENCES
AVSC (1989) *Report on Latin American Regional Postpartum Workshop*, Association for Voluntary Surgical Contraception, Mexico City.

Bulut, A. and Molzan, J. (1993) *A Diagnostic Study for Postpartum Family Planning Service Delivery in Istanbul: A Final Report.*

Castadot, R.G., Sivin, I., Reys, P., *et al.* (1975) *The International Postpartum Family Planning Program: Eight years of experience.* Reports on Population/Family Planning, No. 18.

Coeytaux, F. (1989) *Celebrating Mother and Child on the Fortieth Day: The Sfax, Tunisia, Postpartum Program.* Quality/Calidad/Qualité, No. 1, The Population Council, New York.

CPFH (1989) *Operations Research Program, Five-Year Report.* DPE-3030-A-00-4094, October 1, 1984 to September 30, 1989. Center for Population and Family Health, School of Public Health, Columbia University, New York.

Diaz, S. (1992) *Integrating Postpartum Health Care and Family Planning: The Chilean Experience.* Paper presented at the Population Council Seminar *Rethinking Postpartum Health Care,* New York.

Elias, C. (1993) *A Puzzle of Will: Responding to Reproductive Tract Infections in the Context of Family Planning Programs.* Paper presented at The Africa Operations Research and Technical Assistance Project Conference, Nairobi.

Fall, M. (1992) *Integrating Mother and Child Health Services in Senegal.* Paper presented at the Population Council Seminar *Rethinking Postpartum Health Care,* New York.

Faundes, A. (1992) *Overview of Service Integration: Challenges and Possibilities.* Paper presented at the Population Council Seminar *Rethinking Postpartum Health Care,* New York.

Kennedy, K.I., Rivera, R., and McNeilly, A.S. (1989) Consensus statement on the use of breastfeeding as a planning method. *Contraception,* **39**(5): 447–496.

Mensch, B. (1992) *Overview of the Timing Dilemma.* Paper presented at the Population Council Seminar *Rethinking Postpartum Health Care,* New York.

Potter, R.G., Masnick, G., Stephen, and Gendell, M. (1973) Post amenorrheic versus postpartum strategies of contraception. *Demography,* **10**(1): 99–112.

Potter, R.G, Kobrin, F.E., and Langsten, R.L. (1979) Evaluating acceptance strategies for timing of postpartum contraception. *Studies in Family Planning,* **10**(5): 151–160.

Rogow, D. (1992) *Afterword: Programmatic issues at the seminar on Rethinking Postpartum Health Care.* Paper presented at the Population Council Seminar *Rethinking Postpartum Health Care,* New York.

Taylor, H.C. and Berelson, B. (1970) Maternity and family planning as a world program. In: Zatuchni, G. (ed.), *Postpartum Family Planning: A Report on the International Program.* McGraw-Hill, New York.

Tom, S. (1992) *Two Paradigms of Maternity Health Care.* Paper presented at Population Council Seminar *Rethinking Postpartum Health Care,* New York.

Townsend, J. and Tolbert, K. (1990) *Programmatic Issues and Concerns Surrounding Postpartum Contraception.* Paper presented at the International Conference on Postpartum Contraception.

Winikoff, B. (1992) *What is Postpartum Reproductive Health Care?* Opening remarks at the Population Council Seminar *Rethinking Postpartum Health Care,* New York.

Winikoff, B. and Mensch, B. (1991) Rethinking postpartum family planning. *Studies in Family Planning,* **22**(5): 294–307.

Zatuchni, G.I. (1970) *Postpartum Family Planning: A Report on an International Program,* McGraw-Hill, New York.

CHAPTER

7

More than Pregnancy Care: The Role of the *Matrona* in Women's Reproductive Health in Chile

Susan F. Murray and **Delia Susana Veraguas Segura**

Chile is a thin stretch of land encompassing everything from desert in the north to Antarctic conditions in the south, with a population of around 13 million. The country is undergoing considerable demographic and epidemiological transition.

The maternal mortality ratio has dropped dramatically in the past 30 years, from 299/100,000 live births in 1960 to 41/100,000 in 1989. Fertility rates have fallen from 3.5% to 2.3%, life expectancy at birth has increased from 58 years in 1960 to 72 years in 1990, and infant mortality has decreased from 136/1000 live births in 1960 to 14.4/1000 in 1991 (Jiménez, 1993).

Health care in Chile is provided at primary, secondary, and tertiary levels, and the midwife, the *matrona*, is involved in all of these, although the roles she plays within them are quite distinct. The *matrona* is named in the *Código Sanitario* (Health Code) as the person authorized by law to care for women in pregnancy and birth, and for the new-born; also, as in dentistry and medicine, midwifery is a *profesión libre* – a profession in its own right. Legally, therefore, the midwife can attend her own private patients, although the majority of midwives work within the state sector, or within a doctor's clinic or hospital in the private sector. As in other countries, midwifery in Chile traditionally focused on pregnancy and delivery care, but over the past three decades the *matrona* has also been pivotal in expanding primary health care (PHC) provision. It is this extension of the *matrona*'s role to include many new areas of women's health care which is particularly interesting, and which we explore in this chapter.

THE POLITICAL AND ECONOMIC BACKGROUND
The figures quoted above indicate an impressive health status for a lower middle-income country with a per capita income of $US2500; indeed, Chile has a long tradition of social policies that address educational and health needs. The literacy

rate is 94% and those aged 15 years and above have an average of 10 years of schooling, both women and men. Most of the population has access to safe drinking water (98.5%), and 83% have access to sewerage systems, although less than 6% of the sewage is treated (Jiménez, 1993).

From 1924 there has been health-care provision for workers, and since 1952 Chile has had a national health service, which prioritized mother and child health (MCH) and primary care. The National System of Health Services includes 181 hospitals and 1311 facilities offering MCH care throughout the country (210 urban, 107 rural general clinics, and 994 rural health posts). The 62,000 health workers employed in the system include just over 2000 professional *matronas* (Herrera-Moore, 1988).

However, the public health care system in Chile has also faced problems in recent times. While historically it has been among the most advanced in Latin America, it was affected badly by monetarist policies during the years of the Pinochet military dictatorship (1973–1989). After the military coup in 1973 there was an austere economic reform programme with dramatic reductions in the public sector budget and a privatization drive. Health spending fell by 40% between 1973 and 1987 (Jiménez, 1993). The recession of 1982–1983 resulted in a spending freeze, and all the hospitals were ordered not to fill vacancies. A survey carried out by the College of Midwives in 1984 showed that by then nearly 50% of all trained midwives were either unemployed or not working as midwives (Anderson, 1989). Unsurprisingly, this resulted in a deterioration in care and depersonalized treatment from the hard-pressed staff who remained.

The College of Midwives came under some attack during the dictatorship. In 1981 its role in training was removed by the government as part of the liberalization of the employment market under the regime's economic policy. In 1982 membership of the association ceased to be obligatory for midwives, and it lost its control over ethical standards. This was a time in which many had to keep their heads down to survive, but by the late 1980s the College began to take a more active stand on the right to health and health care. Its 1988 conference noted "the lack of an adequate infrastructure for primary health care in the country, the growing pressure on the secondary sector and the lack of co-ordination between the two" (quoted in Anderson, 1989).

The Health Service, the biggest employer in the country, was broken up into 27 regional authorities in 1979, an action justified in terms of 'decentralization', but which destroyed the national framework. As well as this, primary health care and its 14,000 staff were transferred to the municipalities. Inevitably, there were large differences in disposable incomes between the rich and poor municipalities. Since resources from the government did not compensate adequately for this, municipalization actually accentuated the difference in quality of health care available in rich and poor communities (Miranda, 1992).

The biggest problem of all is co-ordination between primary and secondary levels. There is a dislocation between the administration of the PHC sector and of the hospital system; referral between the two systems is often poor and little information is fed back to the referring agent. This dislocation is reflected in the fragmentation of care available to the pregnant woman within the state health services. She receives all her pregnancy and postnatal care from her midwife in the *consultorio* (health centre) or at the health post, but has to go to the hospital for her delivery, attended by different staff. It is only those who can afford private care who can have continuity of carer throughout, and for most of these the principal carer is an obstetrician, not a midwife.

As in many countries, health-sector finance is currently under review, and the private sector is growing. Chile had the oldest social security system in Latin America, and after the integration of the 35 social security institutions in the late 1970s this covered 75% of the population (WHO, 1993). However, with the radical economic changes of the 1980s the health care fund was separated off from the income maintenance fund (unemployment and pensions, etc.), and a growing and important role was given to the private sector in the management of the funds. All those in employment are currently required to take out health insurance, with a premium of at least 7% of their salaries. This can be paid either into FONASA (Fondo Nacional de Salud), which is the the National Health Fund, or into one of the private medical insurance companies, called ISAPREs (Institutos de Salad Previsional). The private medical insurance system now provides cover for 23% of the population. Health care for the uninsured is provided by the Ministry of Health. In principle, every worker can choose any insurance mechanisms. However, access is limited in practice by the cost of the premiums. Only the relatively well-off can afford ISAPRES, the benefits of which are proportional to the amount paid in. Those with higher incomes are very well serviced, but those with lower incomes have poor access to care. An ISAPRES subscriber may have her baby in a private maternity clinic or in the private wing of a state hospital. An uninsured woman will have no option but the local public hospital.

MIDWIFERY TRAINING

Midwifery is one of eight careers offered by the faculties of medicine of the major universities in Chile, and the schools of midwifery are academic units within these faculties. The first *Escuela de Matronas* (midwifery school), in Santiago, was founded in 1834. The government had decided to start a system of state schools to train doctors, pharmacists, and midwives. It was the first midwifery school to be created in Latin America, and a French doctor, Lorenzo Sazie, was contracted by the Chilean government to be its director, as well as to run the clinical obstetrics course for the medical school. Midwifery training took 2 years, and much emphasis was laid on the moral values which must be possessed by those who dedicated themselves to this activity (Universidad de Chile Facultad de Medicina Carrera de Obstetricia y Puericultura, 1994). Once the first intake graduated in 1836, the government decreed that for those towns in which there were graduates of the midwifery school, only they were permitted to help women in labour (Chang Hernández, 1994).

The path of midwifery training did not, however, run entirely smoothly from then on. The courses were highly dependent on the availability of a director to run and teach them. Epidemics of puerperal fever caused many maternal deaths and resulted in the closure of the maternity wards on several occasions, with suspension of the courses. However, these were temporary obstacles and by 1896 midwifery training had acquired university status when it became the responsibility of the Faculty of Medicine. In 1913, it combined with the *Escuela de Puericultura* to become the *Escuela de Obstetricia y Puericultura* (Universidad de Chile Facultad de Medicina Carrera de Obstetricia y Puericultura, 1994).

In 1930 the course was expanded to 3 years, including a year of work on the maternity unit. Over the next 20 years the entry qualifications were raised and studies expanded to included bacteriology, immunology, pharmacology, and social medicine. Although doctors ran the midwifery school, midwives collaborated in the planning of the studies and in clinical supervision, and their appointment as instructors also began. It was not until the university reforms in 1968 that the first midwife director was appointed to the University of Chile's *Escuela de Obstetricia y Puericultura*.

Midwifery schools were also being created in other regions of the country – Valparaiso in 1955, Temuco in 1963, Antofagasta in 1966, and at the Hospital Salvador in 1967. At that time many midwives worked in remote rural areas, training the traditional *partera* (birth attendants) and working almost single-handedly, with little back-up except for a doctor visiting once a month and emergency facilities available only in the cities. These midwives were often the first professionals to arrive in remote areas, so they had to learn to carry out external cephalic version, manual removal of the placenta, and forceps deliveries, even though these were not part of their formal training as *matronas*. The training schools still tended to be geared to the needs of practice in urban communities, but as recognition of their crucial function in remote areas grew, training placements in rural areas were given more emphasis from 1967.

Professional care in childbirth stood at 18.5% in 1938, but rose to 57.3% during the next 20 years. By 1978, 89.6% of births were attended by professionals and since the second half of the 1980s the rate has remained between 97 and 98.8% (Chang Hernández, 1993). This seems to have played an important part in bringing down the maternal mortality ratio. The neonatal mortality rate also declined from 33.9/1000 live births in 1962 to 9.9/1000 by 1985 (Herrera-Moore, 1988). All health posts have equipment for emergency deliveries, and the rural ones have telephones or radios. The clinics have an ambulance to collect and transfer women in labour. The goal has been for all births to take place within health institutions.

MIDWIVES' WORK IN HOSPITALS

At the secondary level, midwives work in both specialized health centres and hospitals. They care for women in labour and attend 80% of the deliveries. Midwives also run the gynaecology wards, with a team that may include medical, surgical, and oncology nurses. Gynaecology has been included in the midwifery curriculum since 1974, when the Ministry of Health delegated gynaecological nursing-care functions to midwives.

At the tertiary level, midwives also work in the care of high-risk obstetrics in a doctor-led team, and are the day-to-day administrators and care providers in neonatal intensive-care units. There are four levels of hospital, the most basic being level four. At this level, typically, there is one midwife on duty each shift who, with other auxiliary personnel, cares for women in labour. Anyone with complications would be transferred to a referral hospital.

Labour-ward care tends to be very medical. There has been little mainstream interest in active birth or natural birth techniques as yet, although these do have some important advocates among both midwifery educationalists and some of the non-government organizations working in women's health (Szewkis and Arroyo, 1985; AFSC, 1991; DOMOS, 1992; Bonilla Gómez, 1994). Such methods are available in a few private clinics.

Labour companions are still not generally allowed in government hospitals, delivery tables have stirrups, and routine episiotomies are still practised. However, the situation is not static. Signs of a change in practice are beginning to emerge; the shaving of pubic hair is no longer routine in many places, and there are successful pilot projects, such as the Hospital 'Van Buren', the largest state hospital in Valparaiso, which modified its labour rooms to allow the presence of companions. There are, however, disturbingly high rates of caesarean section, at almost 29% in the public sector and around 56% in the private sector (Castro, 1994; Ministerio de Salud, 1994). The partograph is widely used, and active management of labour is gaining in popularity in some institutions. An important sign of change, and of humanization of the service, is that the Baby Friendly Hospital Initiative has taken off in recent years. It remains to be seen whether this will be followed by other initiatives to reduce unnecessary intervention in natural processes.

Many of the state hospitals take both public and private patients. The private wings are being enlarged and improved to raise money for the public wings and so that hospitals can be more self-financing. In the private maternity wing the woman's delivery is attended by her private doctor. There are also private clinics and private hospitals in which all obstetric care can be provided to those with the finances to afford it. In this sector the role of the midwife is much reduced; she is an assistant to the obstetrician/gynaecologist (who attends even the normal births), but she can still earn much more doing this than by working in the government sector.

Within the public services wages are lower in the primary health-care sector (where they are determined by the municipality) than in hospitals (where they are set by the Ministry of Health). Hospital midwives can earn twice as much by working night shifts. Working in hospital also has a higher status, as in many countries, presumably because of the orientation to higher technology.

THE MIDWIFE'S WORK WITHIN PRIMARY HEALTH CARE

In Chile, primary health care is the base of a pyramid that offers widespread health surveillance and treatment of simple pathologies, as well as referral to the second and third levels of specialization and hospital care. Primary mother and child health services in Chile cover antenatal care, feeding programmes, early detection of gynaecological and breast cancer, family planning, health education, well-child care, vaccinations, environmental sanitation, and the diagnosis and prevention of sexually transmitted diseases (STDs).

It is actually in the primary care sector that the most interesting and exciting developments in the midwife's role have occurred, and where the potential for the future is most striking.

Chile now has a largely urban population – 83.4% (Colegio Médico de Chile, 1994) – but there are still many scattered communities in remote areas. Rural health posts are staffed by auxiliary nurses, who have had training in rural heath care and who live permanently in the community. These auxiliaries map their villages, identifying households with members at particular health risk (Ringeling and Herrera, 1992). Communities are visited regularly (weekly or monthly, depending on the distance) by the midwife, as well as by the nurse, doctor, and dentist. Rural nursing stations in small communities may be consulting rooms in community halls or classrooms. In the far north and south of Chile people live in extremely isolated conditions, so the midwife's round may involve the use of light aircraft or motorboats to cross the channels and reach the many islands of the south, or four-wheel drive vehicles to reach the villages of the *altiplano*. In its attempt to reduce the inaccessibility of institutional delivery due to distance and transport difficulties, Chile was one of the first countries to use maternity waiting homes near to the hospitals that served rural areas. La Casita in rural Traiguén became, in 1975, the first home in Chile for high-risk pregnant women from the countryside (Levy, 1990).

Small sectors of the population still resist the institutionalization of birth. Of the population in the country's ninth region, 37% are of Mapuche descent. For many Mapuche, the *machi* is still the traditional provider of health care, using a 'hot' and 'cold' model of health care (Oyarce, 1988). These Mapuches still consider birth to be a natural event. Some still use a rope to hold in the squatting position and give birth at home, although most – 81.8% in one study (San Miguel *et al.*, 1987) – attend a health post or *consultorio* for antenatal care. In such communities professional attendance at deliveries is not universal (San Miguel *et al.*, 1987).

At the primary health-care level, the *matrona*'s focus is the promotion and protection of maternal and perinatal health, and she is employed in rural health posts and urban and rural *consultorios* (health centres). Here she provides care that spans much of a woman's life. A typical midwife in the primary health-care sector may work in a rural area of around 11,000 inhabitants, be based in two *consultorios* with two additional rural health posts to visit, and distribute her time between them. She runs the antenatal and postnatal clinics, and is responsible for the care and screening of the new-born for the first 28 days of life, including giving the BCG vaccination.

Since 1980 the *matrona* has also been the professional who performs cervical and breast screening (Lorenzetti Silva, 1994). She also runs the family planning services within the government sector. Indeed, family planning service provision would scarcely exist in Chile without the midwife – 96.4% of contraceptive consultations [oral contraceptive prescription, insertion of intrauterine contraceptive devices (IUCD), advice, and follow-up] were carried out by *matronas* in 1989 (Chang Hernández, 1993).

THE DEVELOPMENT OF FAMILY PLANNING SERVICES

The government family planning services began in the mid-1960s because of pressures from two quarters. Health professionals in Chile were anxious to improve overall maternal and child health status, and were deeply concerned about the high levels of maternal mortality and morbidity resulting from induced abortion. In the early 1960s the abortion rate was officially estimated at 32/1000 women of fertile age, but the true occurrence was believed to be higher (Rosselot and Mardones, 1990). In 1964, 20% of the beds in the maternity services were devoted to abortion complications.

Parallel to this, in the 1950s the United States and other Western powers were becoming concerned about the 'population explosion' in developing countries. It became the major issue of the World Conference on Population in 1954, and resulted in the development of diverse new organizations, including the Population Council which began to develop activities to control population growth in countries such as Chile.

Thus, the Ministry of Health and the Asociación de Protección de la Familia (APROFA) began to introduce family planning services within the MCH programme of the country, and from 1966 until recently USAID has, through APROFA, supplied the Ministry with free contraceptives. Family planning services were incorporated in the women's health programme in 1965, and a core of 300 physicians and midwives were selected for training in family planning methods (IUCD and oral contraceptives only) and education, and then went on to train others in multiplier courses (Kwast, 1991).

During the years of the socialist Allende government, fertility regulation was seen as part of an integrated family health and welfare programme, and some emphasis was given to sex education as part of this. However, with the military coup in September 1973 a restructuring of the health sector began and by 1976 the tone of the family planning service had changed. In 1974 the programme was extended to the north of the country (Delgado, 1976), but although the methods would still be available if requested, there was to be no educational work or promotional work about the services. The dictatorship was pro-natalist, and the programme turned into one that promoted 'responsible parenting'; the new emphasis was on the dignity of motherhood and the 'inalienable right to life of the fetus' from the moment of conception, which was included in the constitution in 1980. Chile is a profoundly Catholic country, and the tenets of the Catholic Church have influenced women's access to reproductive health care in a number of areas. Female sterilization, for example, is difficult to obtain in Chile. It is performed after the third caesarean section, and is also available only to women over 30 years old who have four living children and have tried other methods unsuccessfully (Viel, 1993). The agreement of three specialists is required.

In spite of the limitations on the provision of family planning services, the maternal mortality from abortion was cut from 60/100,000 live births in 1960 to 14/100,000 by 1989, and the total fertility rate fell from 4.7 in 1960 to 2.4 in 1987 (Rosselot and Mardones, 1990). However, when the numbers of midwives and staff to provide contraceptive services were reduced in the economic crisis of the mid-1980s, queues grew longer and women were frequently turned away. Viel (1993) suggests that this may be why, between 1985 and 1990, the number of hospitalizations for abortions actually began to rise again – by nearly 8000 to 44,468, a return to the 1970 levels. The notable decrease in maternal mortality remained, however, due to improvements in medical treatment and antibiotic use.

In 1988 the criminalization of abortion was completed as even therapeutic abortion was prohibited, accompanied by aggressively anti-abortion coverage on the television. This ban, issued by the outgoing military junta, ironically coincided with the news that Chile had ratified the UN Convention Against all Forms of Discrimination Against Women. There were an estimated 150,000 illegal abortions a year being carried out in Chile, that is around 400 a day (SERNAM, 1992), or one for every 2.5 births, and more than 30,000 women are hospitalized each year as a result of complications (IPPF, 1994). It remains the leading cause of maternal death, accounting for about 34% of the total.

OUTREACH

The midwife's extended role in the primary health-care sector does not stop at family planning. She also provides screening and treatment for STDs for both male and female patients, and does the contact tracing. She is authorized to prescribe basic antibiotics. Her remit includes outreach work, such as domiciliary visits to women with high risk pregnancies and to non-attendees at the clinic. She may also visit the mother and new baby postnatally at home before their eighth day return visit to the clinic, to see that all is going well. She may also visit women with positive smear results, who will then be referred to a specialist clinic in the city. She has health education responsibilities and may run antenatal classes after the clinic sessions, as well as providing education for the general population in the waiting room. She may run workshops in the community, in schools, and with the *Centros de Madres*, a community organization for women. She may initiative a local campaign to increase the uptake of cervical smears, which are available to all women over 25 years, or are sexually active every 3 years, or on request, but which are not popular with many women.

The midwife's official working week is 44 hours, for a monthly wage the equivalent of about $US320, but much of the paper work, statistics, and preparation for educational work has to be done at home during evenings and weekends. If there is not enough time or resources to go around, it is often the educational and outreach work that is not done. Clinics are reimbursed for all the activities that they undertake, but domiciliary visits and group education are poorly funded. There are thus 'perverse incentives' to prioritize clinical work and screening in the clinic, for which reimbursement is higher.

ADOLESCENT REPRODUCTIVE HEALTH

One of the recent developments in the Maternal and Perinatal Health Programme has been the emphasis on care specifically for the pregnant adolescent. The initiation of sexual relations at an early age is common in Latin America, but the use of contraceptive methods is very limited. Of course, adolescent pregnancy is not new, but some of its social characteristics have changed from those in previous decades. There have been changes in the patterns of family life, in behavioural norms and sexual attitudes in young people, and in the status of women; all these are reflected in its increased identification as a 'problem'.

Fertility in the age group 10–19 years has declined little between 1960 and 1987, compared with the large reduction in older age groups, probably because of the lack of sex education and family planning services appropriate to the needs of this group (Asociación Chilena de Protección de la Familia, 1991). Relatively, the proportion of children to mothers under 20 years old is increasing; 40,000 births a year are to under 20 year olds, 14% of total births. In 1989, of the 125 maternal deaths in Chile, 16 were adolescents (12.8%) and infant mortality of children of adolescent mothers is higher than the national average, at 30/1000 live births as compared with 20.5/1000 (SERNAM, 1992). In Chile the unmarried pregnant adolescent is often rejected both by her family group and by the father of her child (Molina and Romero, 1985). Also, the higher frequency of perinatal complications among pregnant adolescents seems to be associated with ignorance and with little or no medical care.

Since 1980 there has been increased interest in adolescent pregnancy, particularly because of the ground-breaking work of CEMERA, the Centro de Medicina Reproductiva del Adolescente of the University of Chile. Almost all the hospitals and *consultorios* in Chile now run a programme of *Atención de la Embarazada y Madre Adolescente*, usually involving a midwife, social worker, and, increasingly, a psychologist.

Special antenatal groups for pregnant adolescents are gaining in popularity, and many midwives are now attending training courses in this field.

Until 1985 there was no mention in official documents of fertility regulation for adolescents, unsurprising perhaps, given the government's emphasis on the family unit. Then, for the first time, because adolescents had been identified as a group at high obstetric risk, prevention of adolescent pregnancy appeared as one of the objectives of the maternal and infant health and family planning programme (Instituto de la Mujer, 1989).

Subsequently, in 1990 an internal document of the Ministry of Health recognized that the risk factors for teenage pregnancy arose fundamentally from 'the psychological and social environment', and that special services were needed for adolescents. After a year-long analysis of Chile's health situation, the Ministry of Health in 1991 formulated a new maternal and child health programme, designed to ensure that all pregnancies would be desired and would occur under optimal conditions. Orientation for responsible parenthood was to be part of the process, and other objectives included reducing the incidence of adolescent pregnancy and of STDs. However, there are still almost no contraceptive services designed and run specifically for young people.

Alongside this, Circular No. 247 of the Ministry of Education (March 1991) instructed that students should be allowed to continue their studies if they married or assumed maternal responsibilities (Galaz, 1994). An increasing number of educational establishments do have policies to allow girls who become pregnant to continue their studies, but the majority do not come back to school after the birth. In one analysis of 650 teenagers, 55.8% were studying when they became pregnant, but by 1 year after the birth only 6.9% had continued with their studies. The mother usually needed to earn a living while a relative cared for their child, and the father abandoned his partner and did not visit his child in 60% of the cases (SERNAM, 1992).

Some midwives are beginning to become involved in sex education in schools, as this is part of the strategy for prevention. By and large this was completely missing from the school curricula in Chile in the 1960s and 1970s. The most that might be hoped for was references to animal reproduction. A programme of family life and sex education was published by the Ministry of Education in 1971 and was tried in some schools, but after the coup in 1973 it was withdrawn. In 1980–1981 the theme returned to the curriculum, but with a strong emphasis on the family, responsible parenting, and child-rearing. Contraception was not covered and premarital sexual relationships went undiscussed (Instituto de la Mujer, 1989). By 1984 there was national concern about the level of STDs, and the Ministry of Health made a declaration about the importance of including a discussion of STDs within sex education. By 1986 'sexuality and love' had been included in sex education in schools, but still only within the context of 'the family' and still with no mention of contraceptive methods (Instituto de la Mujer, 1989).

Even now, in the mid-1990s, sex education is still only carried out in some schools; in others, parents still object or the teachers do not feel adequately prepared to provide it. There are inter-sectoral committees between education and health, at both Ministry and local levels. Some of these work very well and others do not. The more pro-active midwives are beginning to be involved in work in schools, again often with a social worker and psychologist, and student midwives are being involved in this in their community placements. It is likely to be an area of expansion for midwives in the future.

CARE FOR THE OLDER WOMAN

Owing to the demographic transition, the characteristics of Chilean society are changing with proportionately more older people than ever before. People are living longer – life expectancy for women is projected to be 75 years in the period 1995–2000. This may mean a changing emphasis in the future role of the midwife. Such changes have been highlighted and applauded by leading figures in midwifery, who argue that the *matrona*, while still playing her important traditional part in maternal and infant health, should have an increasing role to play in the gynaecological and well-woman care of the older female population (Chang Hernández, 1990; Lorenzetti Silva, 1994).

The pharmaceutical companies were quick to promote hormone replacement therapy (HRT) to the medical profession in Chile, and through them to the female population at large. Midwives do not prescribe HRT, but, with the increasing medicalization of this area of women's lives, they are beginning to provide health education for women in the peri-menopausal period. Workshops are being run in health centres for women in the 40–60 age group, using participative methods. Their aim is to help older women to improve their 'quality of life'.

These new developments are based on the argument that, with the increase in life expectancy for women and the average menopause beginning at between 48 and 51 years, "a third of a woman's life is spent with oestrogen deprivation, the biggest risks of pathology associated with the end of ovarian function being coronary heart disease, osteoporosis, and emotional problems" (Lagos and Navarro, 1994).

One might be a little dismayed at this portrayal of what is, after all, a perfectly normal life process as a deficiency or 'deprivation'. However, this 'midwifery perspective' of the menopause does, at least, argue that oestrogen therapy is not the only thing that an older woman needs, to come to terms with the changed, often diminished, role. Its proponents argue that women need to acquire knowledge about the menopause, risk of pathologies, health promotion (cancer of the cervix, breast cancer), and personal growth so as to preserve their quality of life and to care for themselves.

Certainly, the supportive function of such workshops may be considerable. In a recent paper in the College of Midwives' journal reporting on a series of such workshops in Temuco, the organizers describe how the groups of women gave support to each other, sharing their sensation of loss, emptiness, and of having lived solely for the family. They expressed their need to change and to develop themselves as women and as people, and particularly wanted to know more about sexuality and psychological change (Lagos and Navarro, 1994).

There is rising interest in *autocuidado* – self care – among health promoters and health-care providers in Chile. For many years the service was dominated by the notion that health was in the hands of the health professional, but now there are some attempts to shake of this messianic role and to acknowledge that it is the woman who cares for herself, her body, and her health (and that of her family), and that she should be encouraged to have confidence in herself. Many midwives still find this difficult – like doctors, they have been the 'experts' for so long. However, the increased contact and work with other groups, such as social workers, is gradually helping them to see things in different ways.

CHALLENGES FOR THE FUTURE

The *matrona* in Chile has many functions. She provides antenatal and postnatal care, family planning services, gynaecological screening, health education, care in childbirth and to the new-born, care of obstetric and gynaecological morbidity, and health promotion in the family and the community. The reasons for midwifery becoming so integral to the provision of these services in Chile are, no doubt, partly historical and partly economic. The historical reasons for midwifery, rather than nursing, taking on these roles probably derive from the former's (perceived) parallel relationship to medicine, which traditionally includes both obstetrics and gynaecology in one speciality. The economics of employing midwives (even university-trained midwives), rather than doctors, to perform these functions are self-explanatory. Furthermore, one of the characteristics of the Chilean midwife has been her commitment, her social conscience – in spite of low wages and long hours. However, such goodwill should not be overexploited. In so far as there is any opposition among midwives themselves towards the further extension of their responsibilities, it derives from being asked to take on more and more activities, but with the same official hours of work and the same low salaries.

As a profession midwifery is competing with both medicine and nursing for space and for status. Midwifery training has continued to increase in length and sophistication over the years. In 1974, training was expanded to 4 years and, significantly, from that time men as well as women were accepted as student midwives. During the 1980s the curriculum was modified to include administration and health planning, and from 1990, social science and research methods.

At present midwives in Chile are technically very competent. In the past 5 or 6 years, midwives have become involved in conducting their own research, holding workshops and conferences at which they present their own work. There are still relatively few midwives with postgraduate qualifications, and midwives are rarely in a position to influence policy or to form it. The pyramidal hierarchy within health care still has the medical profession firmly holding the power.

The semi-private Catholic University and the University of Valparaiso tried to incorporate midwifery within a wider nursing profession, by designing an *enfermera matrona* (nurse midwife) qualification that took 5 years. They were fiercely opposed in this by prominent members of the College of Midwives, who felt strongly that there is a need to protect midwifery as a separate profession. The course went ahead, because it was felt that such a joint qualification would be particularly suitable for work in rural and marginal communities (and would presumably remove the necessity and expense of employing both a nurse and a midwife to cover MCH services). However, the graduates from these courses reported that they did not feel that the broader training equipped them to deal adequately with birth in isolated communities. Almost all of the *enfermera matronas* who qualified went into conventional nursing posts. Taking this into account the University of Valparaiso plans to separate the two careers again in 1996.

At the end of 1993 a new study plan was approved for the midwifery training run by the University of Chile, one of the country's largest universities. The new qualification will be a *Licenciatura en Obstetricia y Puericultura*, with an increase from 4 to 5 years of study. The University will also initiate a parallel programme to enable qualified midwives to reach this level. The significance of this title is that it can only be conferred by a university, not by any other institute, thus effectively preserving the midwifes status as a university-trained professional. To be a *licenciada* will signify greater autonomy, and will open up more opportunities for midwives to become involved in academic activities and in research, to become specialists in areas such as neonatology, or go on to Masters or Doctorates in a field such as public health. The vision of the new midwifery professional is one capable of continually incorporating new advances into her work and of being creative in the development of Ministry of Health policies.

These developments are particularly notable when one considers the erosion and virtual destruction of the midwifery profession that has occurred in other Latin American countries, such as Argentina and Brazil (Faundes and Cecatti, 1989; Szmoisz and Vartabedian, 1992). But such professionalization strategies are inevitably double-edged. On the one hand, increasing professionalization may succeed in obtaining the space, status, and intellectual forum necessary for midwifery not only to survive, but to develop and to become more powerful. On the other hand, there may be risks. The danger, present in any country where increased professionalization is in progress, is that a new career ladder which rewards specialization and academic achievement may prove to be a greater motivator to the next generation of midwives than any 'old-fashioned' notions of public service. If that happens, the MCH services would lose one of its greatest assets, midwives dedicated to work in unglamorous rural and poor urban communities.

The challenges facing the midwifery profession in Chile in its next phase are many. Years of inflexibility and lack of questioning under a military dictatorship had left the profession without much contact with the outside world. Childbirth-care practices have become heavily institutionalized and have changed little in 20 years. Because of the economic austerity programme, the technical and administrative processes have deteriorated and many of the protocols and procedures are old-fashioned. Queues, long waiting lists, and delays in referral pose real practical problems (Colegio Médico de Chile, 1994). The strong emphasis on interventionist procedures in obstetric practice requires urgent review, and the lack of continuity of care through pregnancy and delivery to postpartum needs to be challenged.

On top of this, with the return to democracy, the public sector is in some turmoil. The 16 years of containing costs and not investing have led to a crisis that surfaced with the return to elected government in 1990. There was a health workers' strike within months and soon after doctors took repeated industrial action. Wages have been increased by 35%, but are still low. World Bank and Inter-American Development Bank loans have been accepted to improve the infrastructure, and the World Bank is currently assisting in a health-sector reform project whose stated objective is to "achieve a proper private–public mix for the whole country" (Jiménez, 1993). It still remains to be seen what a 'proper mix' might be.

On the other hand, there have been some remarkable achievements in spite of very difficult times. In the primary health-care sector the midwifery profession has been pivotal in whole new areas of reproductive health-care provision for women. The Maternal and Perinatal Programme is now being renamed the Women's Health

Programme in recognition of its broad scope and emphasis on a women's complete life span and on the impact of gender roles on health.

A working group of midwives has been given the responsibility of developing the guidelines on how this programme should be implemented (Revista Colegio de Matronas, 1994). The extended role lays increasing emphasis on early screening, prevention, and community health promotion. The approach is increasingly biosocial, with much emphasis on participation of the user groups in tackling health problems. New and challenging skills are being required of the midwife. Her broadening public-health role, combined with that of the carer of individual women with individual needs, will make the progress of the Chilean midwife of international interest in the coming years.

ACKNOWLEDGEMENTS

The authors wish to give their sincere thanks to the following midwives for their time, experience, help, and knowledge in the research for this chapter: Nelly Chang Hernández, Hilda Bonilla Gómez, María Filomena Fuentes Jeraldino, Elba Luna Rojas, Gabriela Jauregui Millán, Leticia Lorenzetti Silva, Margarita Moreno, Ivelise Segovia, and M. Solange Valenzuela.

The responsibility for the views expressed in this chapter, however, remains ours alone.

REFERENCES

AFSC (1991) *El Parto Sin Temor, una experiencia con mujeres embarazadas de sectores marginales.* American Friends Service Committee, Chile.

Anderson, F. (1989) Chilean midwifery under the jackboot. *Nursing Times,* **85**(31): 74–75.

Asociación Chilena de Protección de la Familia (1991) Salud materna y perinatal. *Boletín de APROFA,* **27**(1–12): 1–21.

Bonilla Gómez, H. (1994) Técnicas apropriadas para la atención del parto. *Revista Colegio de Matronas,* **2**(1): 4–7.

Castro, S.R. (1994) La cesárea: Necesidad o abuso? *Revista Colegio de Matronas,* **2**(1): 37–42.

Chang Hernández, N. (1990) Modelo Operacional Para Desarrollo de un Sistema Curricular – Formación del Profesional Matrona. *X Jornadas Chilenas de Salud Publica.* Universidad de Chile Facultad de Medicina Escuela de Salud Publica Ministerio de Salud, Santiago.

Chang Hernández, N. (1993) La matrona en la atención de salud materna y neonatal. *Revista Colegio de Matronas,* **1**(1): 16–23.

Chang Hernández, N. (1994) Diálogo con la historia 160 años de la Escuela de Obstetricia. *Revista Colegio de Matronas,* **2**(1): 32–36.

Colegio Médico de Chile (1994) Proyecto de Salud para Chile. *Cuadernos Médico Sociales,* **35**: 5–55.

Delgado, I.G. (1976) Needs for training personnel in medical and clinical activities: a Chilean experience. In: Sanhueza, H. and Jaimes, R. (eds) *Contraceptive Progress in Latin American and the Caribbean.* Proceedings of IPPF/WHR 2nd Regional Medical Seminar, Nov. 1975, IPPF, New York, pp 52–57.

DOMOS (1992) *Una Nueva Vida Comienza: Guía para la mujer embarazada.* DOMOS: Centro de Desarollo de la Mujer, Santiago.

Faundes, A. and Cecatti, J.G. (1993) Which policy for caesarean sections in Brazil? An analysis of trends and consequences. *Health Policy and Planning,* **8**(1): 33–42.

Galaz, J. (1994) Aulas abiertas a las embarazadas. *La Nación*, 17th August, Santiago, p. 10.

Herrera-Moore, M. (1988) Atención primaria en salud materno infantil. *Revista Chilena de Obstetricia y Ginecologia*, **53**(5): 301–309.

Instituto de la Mujer (1989) *Las Políticas de Planificación Familiar y Educación Sexual en Chile*. Resumen 1, Instituto de la Mujer Area de la Salud, Santiago.

IPPF (1994) Chilean abortion law harmful to women's health. *Open File*, IPPF, February, p. 9.

Jiménez, J. (1993) Re-establishing health care in Chile. *British Medical Journal*, **307**: 729–730.

Kwast, B.E. (1991) Shortage of midwives: the effect on family planning. *IPPF Medical Bulletin*, **25**(3): 1–3.

Lagos, P. X. and Navarro, H. N. (1994) Estrategias educativas para la mujer perimenopausica. *Revista Colegio de Matronas*, **2**(1): 11–14.

Levy, S. (1990) Digno Stagno y la casa de la embarazada rural. *Enfoques en Atención Primaria*, **5**(2): 33–38.

Lorenzetti Silva, L. (1994) Rol de la matrona en la menopausia y el climaterio. *Revista Colegio de Matronas*, **2**(2): 15–21.

Ministerio de Salud Depto. de Coordinación e Informatica (1994) Información estadística de prestaciones ortogadas a beneficios de la ley 18.469 en sus modalidades de libre elección e institucional y sistema de ISAPRE, Chile 1986–1993.

Miranda, R.E. (1992).Cobertura, Eficiencia y Equidad en el Area de Salud en America Latin. *Estudios Públicos*, **46**: 163–248.

Molina, R. and Romero, M.I. (1985) Adolescent pregnancy: the Chilean Experience. In: *Health of Adolescents and Youths in the Americas*. Scientific Publication No. 489, PAHO, Washington, DC, pp 194–205.

Oyarce, P.A.M. (1988) La Salud entre los Mapuches. *Experiencias*, **3**: 1–44.

Revista Colegio de Matronas (1994) Promocion y prevencion: Dos pilares en el programa de Salud de la Mujer. *Revista Colegio de Matronas*, **2**(2): 27–30.

Ringeling, I. and Herrera, G. (1992) Chile's rural nurses. *World Health*, **Sept–Oct**: 8–9.

Rosselot, J. and Mardones, F. (1990) Salud de la familia y paternidad responsable: la experiencia de Chile 1965–1988. *Revista Medica de Chile*, **118**(3): 330–338.

San Miguel, G., Rubilar, C., and Echeverria, V. (1987) Parto Domiciliario. *VII Jornadas de Salud Pública*. Universidad de Chile Facultad de Medicina Escuela de Salud Pública Ministerio de Salud, Santiago.

SERNAM (1992) Embarazo en adolescentes. *Revista Mujer Servicio Nacional de la Mujer*, **1**(3): 10–11.

Szewkis, D. and Arroyo, J.M. (1985) Parto natural: Asumiendo la maternidad. *Psicosexualidad, Revista Chilena de Sexualidad*, **2**(3): 39–43.

Szmoisz, S. and Vartabedian, R. (1992) Midwives: professionals in their own right. *World Health Forum*, **13**: 291–294.

Universidad de Chile Facultad de Medicina Carrera de Obstetricia y Puericultura (1994) *160 Años de la Carrera de Obstetricia y Puericultura 1834–1994*. Universidad de Chile Facultad de Medicina Carrera de Obstetricia y Puericultura, Santiago.

Viel, B.(1993) Chile - the need for reform. *Planned Parenthood Challenges*, **1**: 12–13.

WHO (1993) *Evaluation of Recent Changes in the Financing of Health Services*. WHO Technical Report Series 829, WHO, Geneva

CHAPTER
8

The Right to Know: Women and their Traditional Birth Attendants

Maureen Minden and **Marta J. Levitt**

INTRODUCTION

It is our contention that all women should have access to information about their health in child-bearing, and to have supportive care from someone who understands their needs within the context of their everyday life. In many developing countries this role can be fulfilled best by the indigenous village midwife.

In recent years, however, this central role of the traditional midwife has become obscured in the debate around the prevention of maternal mortality. We argue here that this has occurred because the prevailing perspective of many writers and policy advisors is based on a far too narrow 'crisis management' approach. The current debate on the role and training of traditional birth attendants (TBAs) is reviewed in this chapter, and a practical framework for TBA services in developing countries is suggested.

TBAs: A NATURAL RESOURCE

The value of village midwives as a local maternal health resource was recognized as early as the 1920s (Population Report, 1980; Manglay-Maglacas, 1990). By the 1970s and 1980s training of TBAs had become an integral component of 'mother and child health' programmes, but their role was overshadowed by the international aid community's focus on child survival. This focus continued even after the Alma Ata international conference in 1978, which marked the shift to an integrated primary health-care approach.

Women's health needs were officially recognized at the Safe Motherhood Conference in Nairobi, Kenya, in 1987. The Safe Motherhood Initiative was launched with the overall goal of reducing maternal mortality and morbidity, and the roles that trained TBAs might play in women's health care received renewed interest.

In less-developed countries, TBAs remain the major provider of care for child-bearing women at the community level. The vast majority of women (73%) in the least-developed countries and 45% in developing countries deliver without the assistance of any trained birth attendant, compared to only 2% of child-bearing women in developed countries (UNICEF, 1993). In developing countries, the TBA is likely to be the most immediate source of maternity care.

In the past decade, research on birth attendants has revealed a diversity of traditional roles. In some societies it is recognized that one person may be needed to give support during labour and another needed to cut the cord and give care after delivery (Jeffery *et al.*, 1984; Levitt, 1988). Some women have become TBAs or lay midwives through apprenticeship. A mother-in-law, by tradition, may be the one responsible for her extended family or a woman may become a birth assistant after first being called upon for help by sisters or friends. Recognition of this diversity led to the previously universal definition of TBA being replaced with a range of definitions (WHO, 1992b).

Training of TBAs in community health has expanded over the past 10 years to include immunization, identification and treatment of diarrhoea and acute respiratory infection, and community-based distribution of oral rehydration therapy (ORT) packets and safe birth kits. Furthermore, areas are included which previously were considered to be in conflict with the role of the TBA (e.g., family planning counselling). While initially the trained TBA appeared to be a natural resource for safe motherhood activities at the community level, later her training and role became controversial.

THE CONTROVERSY: CRISIS MANAGEMENT VERSUS COMMUNITY DEVELOPMENT

At its outset, the Safe Motherhood Initiative had a broad and inter-sectoral base for action. The aim was "to enhance the quality and safety of girls' and women's lives through the adoption of a combination of health and non-health strategies" (WHO, 1991). Factors outside the health sector that have contributed to reduced maternal morbidity and mortality rates include:

- Reforms and improved enforcement of laws relating to age at marriage, compulsory education for girls, contraception, and abortion.

- Increased female literacy rates.

- Improved status and empowerment of women.

- Reductions in fertility as a result of better access to modern methods of contraception and safe abortion.

However, when prioritization of safe motherhood interventions began, there was pressure to situate maternal health services in medical centres and priority was given to interventions whose effects showed immediate and visible reductions in maternal mortality (Maine, 1991; WHO, 1992a). The focus then narrowed further to the management of obstetric emergencies within health facilities. When 'lives saved per dollar spent' (estimated cost per death prevented) became the indicator, and 'seven hypothetical programme models' were examined, health centres and rural hospitals were found to be the most cost-effective. Family planning, care in pregnancy, and TBA training, in that order, were found to be the least cost-effective (Maine, 1992).

Research literature on health programme implementation at the community level and the safest place of birth highlight the fallibility of sole dependence on hospitals and doctors (Fathalla, 1987; Ransome-Kuti, 1992; Timyan *et al.*, 1992; Feuerstein, 1993; Minden, 1993, 1995; Walsh *et al.*, 1994). This literature has been largely ignored, however.

Positions have become polarized between those who have a crisis management perspective and those with a community-health development perspective. As has happened in Western countries, those promoting hospital and/ or medical solutions tend to be from the medical profession and its supporting industries, such as drug and medical technology companies. They are powerful, high status, and high profile and are able to attract funding. The critical issues from the crisis management perspective are interventions that reduce maternal mortality from obstetric emergencies, so the focus is on the development of medical facilities that offer surgery, blood transfusion services, and drugs.

The critical issues from the community-health development perspective relate to women's health and access to health care in the context of her everyday life. Economic status, education, social status, the right to make decisions and act on them, access to food, and health status are viewed as interwoven. A multitude of factors may prevent a woman from taking advantage of health care services, even when they are accessible geographically (Fathalla, 1987; Timyan *et al.*, 1992; Minden, 1995). Community development approaches to maternal health therefore link health service provision with activities such as water and sanitation programmes, female literacy classes, income generation and empowerment projects, nutrition, and agricultural programmes.

Both approaches have implications for the training and role of TBAs. Advocates of the crisis management approach see the focus of TBA training and her subsequent role as confined essentially to her connection with obstetric emergencies. The community development approach ascribes the TBA a broader role linked with many dimensions of women's health and well-being (see *Figures 8.1* and *8.2*).

A REALISTIC MANDATE FOR THE TRAINED TBA

As indigenous care givers, village midwives provide culturally appropriate care. However, they may unwittingly contribute to morbidity or mortality through carrying out dangerous practices, such as unsafe abortions and/or genital mutilation using unhygienic techniques and equipment, or by giving wrong advice. An important reason for involving the traditional midwife in the formal health-care system is to improve her health-promoting skills.

With some education, even an illiterate local midwife can learn and pass on new skills and ideas to her community. However, she remains bound by the resources available to her and, while training enables her to put safe mother and new-born care principles into practice, the extent of her role is limited by the realities of her work environment. A framework which indicates what the trained TBA can do in her own practice without medical back-up; what she can do when she has access to and support from health care services; and what she can do as a community member in addition to her work as a practitioner is shown on pages 107–108.

Community health development perspective	Crisis management perspective
1. Women's health is integrally bound up with the political, economic, and socio-cultural realities of their lives.	1. Women's health problems are essentially mechanical, i. e. biophysical and/or biochemical, and can be managed with technical solutions that function independently from other dimensions of their lives.
2. Women, including those who are poor and illiterate, can identify health problems and prioritize needs relevant to their daily lives.	2. International medical experts with a global perspective are the people best qualified to identify women's health problems, and determine points of intervention and appropriate management (Wong, 1992).
3. Women have the right to information about their own bodies, reproduction, and health as well as the right to accessible and acceptable care (Boston Women's Health Collective, 1989; Ehrenricht and English, 1979). Accessibility goes beyond the issue of distance and includes perceived needs, decision-making dynamics, perceived quality of care, trust and familiarity with provider and health care setting, and remuneration to provider (Timyan et al., 1992; Minden, 1994).	3. The medical model of health and disease, with its highly trained professionals and sophisticated technologies, is universally desirable and the most effective approach to safe motherhood (Brims and Griffiths, 1992).
4. Responsibility for health lies with the individual woman, her family, and the community.	4. Responsibility for women's health lies with highly trained professionals. Child-bearing women are viewed as 'patients' or 'clients' who passively require care.
5. Without access to information, women do not automatically seek help from the formal health-care system.	5. Symptomatic women will automatically seek help from the formal medical system.
6. In all communities, there are indigenous care givers to whom women turn for advice and help, who, with additional training, can play a significant rolein maternal health programmes (Levitt, 1993; SWACH, 1992).	6. There is very little that indigenous care providers can do to reduce maternal mortality, even when trained, since obstetric emergencies require surgery, blood transfusion services, and drugs (Maine, 1991).
7. Maternal health programmes require a broad and inter-sectoral approach involving a range of interventions that deal with long-term issues and preventive measures, as well as with crisis management.	7. Safe motherhood is essentially a matter of obstetric emergencies and curative capability.
8. The main goal of a maternal health programme is to reduce maternal morbidity and mortality by improving the health and well-being both of women and of their new-borns.	8. The main goal of a maternal health and/or safe motherhood programme is to reduce maternal mortality from obstetric emergencies.

Figure 8.1 Assumptions underlying the maternal health and safe motherhood debate.

Community health development perspective	Crisis management perspective
1. The training of TBAs is crucial to maternal health efforts at the community level.	1. The training of TBAs is not cost-effective when calculated in terms of the estimated cost of maternal deaths prevented in hospital (Maine, 1992).
2. The trained TBA can facilitate the natural process of child-bearing through supportive and preventive measures, and limited crisis management.	2. The role of a trained TBA is limited to avoiding dangerous practices, recognizing complications, and referring promptly, accompanying women with complications to hospital and reporting to medical staff, medically treating anaemia with iron and folate, giving anti-malarials, and conducting clean deliveries.
3. The trained TBA plays a key role in identifying problems and encouraging the use of referral facilities during emergencies. She is an important liaison between the community and the formal health care system.	3. There is little a trained TBA can do in obstetric emergencies beyond referral and possibly administering oxytocics to limit postpartum haemorrhage from hypotonic uterine action.

Figure 8.2 Implications for training and the role of TBAs.

A practical framework for services provided by a trained TBA

THE TRAINED TBA IN HER OWN PRACTICE
The trained TBA can provide important advice, as she will be able to:

- Advise pregnant women and their families on which locally available foods are important to eat and encourage increased caloric intake.
- Explain the relationship between the eating patterns of the mother and the well-being of the mother and of her growing baby.
- Encourage the family to prepare a clean place and necessary items for the delivery.
- Advise on good hygienic practices for the postpartum mother and new-born.

The trained TBA can use preventive practices during delivery, as she will be able to:

- Conduct cleaner deliveries by arranging for a clean place for delivery, washing her hands before assisting the delivery and/or cord cutting, and sterilizing equipment or using pre-packaged home delivery kits.
- Instruct the mother to empty her bladder at regular intervals to facilitate descent of the fetus, delivery of the placenta, and contraction of the uterus to arrest blood loss.
- Direct the mother in slow delivery of the baby's head to minimize perineal trauma.
- Clear the baby's mouth and nose and wipe the baby's eyes.
- Dry the baby after delivery and ensure that it is kept warm.
- Encourage immediate and exclusive breastfeeding.
- Massage the uterus to stimulate contraction if bleeding occurs.

The trained TBA will not use unsafe practices. For example, she:

- Does not insert any object, substance, or her hand into the vagina for any reason.
- Does not push down on or bind the abdomen during labour.
- Does not instruct the woman to push before the baby's head is visible at the vulva.
- Does not pull on any part of the baby during delivery, or on the cord during delivery of the placenta.
- Does not apply any substance to a tear.
- Does not induce abortion nor perform any type of female genital mutilation

The trained TBA can manage certain limited complications, as she will be able to:

- Gently assist delivery of the head without pulling on the baby's body during a breech delivery.
- Instruct the mother to empty her bladder and put the baby to the breast in the case of a retained placenta.
- Instruct the mother to empty her bladder, put the baby to the breast, and massage a hypotonic uterus to stimulate contraction in the case of postpartum bleeding.
- Resuscitate the new-born who does not breathe spontaneously or is asphyxiated.
- Advise the mother and family on how to care for low birth-weight or premature new-borns.

THE TRAINED TBA AND ACCESSIBLE FORMAL HEALTH-CARE FACILITIES

The trained TBA has knowledge of the available health services and their benefits and acts as a liaison between the community and formal health-care personnel. She refers members of her community to formal health-care facilities when necessary and facilitates their use of these services. She also:

- Encourages women to take advantage of antenatal health services, notably tetanus toxoid immunizations and treatment for anaemia.
- Refers women who show signs of problems in pregnancy or labour.
- Recognizes signs and symptoms of obstetric complications and complications in the new-born and refers these for medical care.
- Is aware of transport facilities and knows how to mobilize them.
- Encourages the use of family planning services.
- Distributes iron and folate tablets, sells or provides disposable delivery kits, and supplies contraceptives.

IN THE COMMUNITY

The trained TBA contributes in ways which go beyond the provision of health services, as she:

- Is proof that illiterate women can learn and put into practice modern, scientific methods.
- Imparts important health messages through formal classes or through informal discussion.

- Is a mediator between modern health-care practices and local traditional practices.
- Is an agent of change, where necessary modifying strongly held practices and beliefs.
- Promotes women's rights to information and active involvement in improving their own health care.
- Introduces and promotes new ideas that can have long-term benefits for health.
- Is a role model for untrained birth attendants.

Realistic indicators for the assessment of trained TBAs

The efficacy and cost-effectiveness of TBA training were brought into question as a reduction in mortality from obstetric emergencies became the sole criterion of safe motherhood efforts. It is clear that to assess a TBA solely on her ability to deal with obstetric emergencies is inappropriate and obscures the impact she can have on making child-bearing healthier and safer in her community. Assessment of the impact of trained TBAs therefore requires indicators that are realistic, appropriate, and measurable.

A long-term planning workshop was held for the national TBA programme in Nepal, and the logical framework approach (NORAD, 1992) was applied to develop appropriate measurable indicators. This is a planning, monitoring, and evaluation tool in which goals and inputs (activities, materials, funds) of a programme are linked directly to specific and measurable outcomes. While these indicators may be applicable to TBA programmes in other countries, contexts vary and we recommend that each country develop indicators appropriate to their situation. In Nepal, the indicators outlined below were included.

COMMUNITY ACCESS TO THE SERVICES OF TRAINED TBAs
This is quantified by the:

- Number of deliveries annually per trained TBA.
- Population per trained TBA as appropriate to the geographic and demographic conditions.
- Distance trained TBAs live from women of reproductive age.

UTILIZATION OF SERVICES PROVIDED BY TRAINED TBAs
This is quantified by the:

- Proportion of pregnant and postpartum women receiving advice from a trained TBA.
- Proportion of pregnant women receiving antenatal care from a trained TBA.
- Proportion of home deliveries conducted by trained TBAs compared to untrained assistants.
- Proportion of women and their new-borns receiving postpartum care from a trained TBA.
- Number of services provided (e.g., antenatal examinations conducted, deliveries attended) per trained TBA.

QUALITY OF SERVICES PROVIDED BY TRAINED TBAs
This is quantified by the:

- Proportion of trained TBAs working according to competency-based standards set in training.
- Changes in TBAs' practices as a result of training, assessed using checklists and interviews with clients.
- Differences in practices of untrained and trained TBAs working under similar circumstances.

CHANGES IN COMMUNITY PRACTICES
- Changes in community birth practices that coincide with TBA training, regardless of who assisted during delivery, are assessed through community surveys.

MATERNAL AND NEONATAL DEATHS AVERTED
These are estimated by the:

- Differences in neonatal and maternal death rates between clients of trained TBAs, clients of untrained TBAs, and national statistics.
- Extent to which trained TBAs save lives as documented through case studies and ethnographic research.

REFERRALS BY TRAINED TBAs
In areas where trained TBAs have access to a formal health institution, a referral system for trained TBAs should be developed and assessed to determine the:

- Proportion of all referrals by trained TBAs.
- Proportion of referrals made appropriately by trained TBAs.
- Proportion of referrals for tetanus toxoid and/or treatment of anaemia made by trained TBAs.
- Proportion of clients of trained TBAs that are fully immunized, are not anaemic, or have been provided with iron and/or folate on a regular basis.
- Effectiveness of TBA referral system, i.e. compliance.

HOSPITAL SERVICES – THEIR ROLE IN MATERNAL HEALTH CARE

It has to be recognized that hospital care for child-bearing women has the potential for harm as well as good. Even with reliable, modern resources hospitals pose risks from incorrect management or unnecessary intervention in pregnancy and childbirth (Richards, 1978; Tew, 1978, 1990). This issue is especially relevant in the context of developing countries, where there is often little in the way of hygienic practice.

In hospitals, there is a temptation to intervene during childbirth when there are technologies on hand and a need to train students in using them. There is also pressure to 'speed things up' because the facilities are filled beyond capacity (Minden, 1995). Antibiotics are often mis-used and can create problems (Pakistan Society of Physicians, 1993; Walsh *et al.*, 1994), as happens with blood transfusions and operative interventions. Hospitals may not even have such resources and, in many remote areas, there are no hospitals.

Nepal, for example, has a population of approximately 20 million of which 90% live rurally. Of the 75 districts, 70 have a district hospital, and each hospital has three posts for doctors. Rarely are all three posts filled, and attracting or keeping trained staff in rural areas is difficult. The hospitals do not have any specialized services and they largely function as out-patient units (Ali, 1991). A recent Ministry of Health report pointed out that "... it appears that district hospitals are not equipped or staffed to handle serious complications and thus must be questioned as a referral source for complicated MCH cases..." (Maskey et al., 1991).

The absence of policies, clinical guidelines, protocols, and monitoring make it impossible to evaluate the quality of care in these hospitals. Furthermore, data are rarely available with which to assess outcome in the days following discharge, as most patients are lost to follow-up. The neonatal mortality rates recorded at maternity hospitals in Nepal include only those deaths that occur during the hospital period although most discharges take place within 24 hours of delivery (Department of Statistics, 1993, personal communication). The maternal mortality rate similarly includes only deaths that occur before discharge from hospital. Sepsis, secondary postpartum haemorrhage, or other causes of morbidity or mortality resulting from mismanagement in hospital, but manifested after discharge, are not officially recorded.

There are socio-cultural implications in defining child-bearing as an abnormal, even pathological, phenomenon. In the West, it has been argued that the medicalization of childbirth has had a destructive socio-cultural and psychological effect on women. Yet the same process is being introduced into developing countries. In the foreign atmosphere of a hospital, rules that prevent a friend or family member being present to give support, bureaucratic procedures that are given precedence over the needs of a woman, and the denigrating attitudes of staff towards poor or illiterate women all contribute to undermining women's confidence.

There is a need to question the cost-effectiveness of hospitals as the top financial priority in health care. Hospitals may absorb more than half of a health-care budget, and yet serve only a small percentage of the population. In Nepal, the 1987–1988 health budget was 4.23% of the national budget, less than the proportion in 1983–1984. Most of this was invested in hospitals in urban centres, where only 7% of the population lived; the greatest portion was spent in the most developed region, where 550 of the 879 doctors, over half of hospital beds, and more than 75 of the 123 hospitals were concentrated (Ali, 1991).

CONCLUSIONS

Misplaced priorities in developing national health-care systems are contributing to the inaccessibility of health information and health care services for the majority of women, including those most in need. The advocates of community health care have been put on the defensive, even though institutional health-care facilities cannot ensure that a child-bearing woman in need of medical assistance will receive adequate or appropriate care. The assumptions underlying each side of the debate concerning priorities in maternal health and/or safe motherhood efforts have not been clarified, nor has the existence of such a debate always been acknowledged. This has led to contradictions and inconsistencies in statements regarding training for TBAs and their subsequent roles, and to the use of inappropriate indicators for evaluating the care they provide.

To ensure that the work of trained TBAs is evaluated justly, realistic indicators should be utilized, and global indicators, such as maternal mortality rates, should be employed with caution. Adequate medical back-up in emergencies may not be accessible even for those within reach of a medical facility. Trained TBAs can provide a means by which village women, who may be illiterate, have access to knowledge about their bodies, health, and childbirth, and access to safer care during child-bearing; TBAs can contribute to the health development of their communities.

REFERENCES

Ali, A. (1991) *Status of Health in Nepal.* Resource Centre for Primary Health Care, Nepal and South–South Solidarity, India.

Boston Women's Health Collective (1989) *Our Bodies, Ourselves.* Penguin Books, London.

Brims, S. and Griffiths, M. (1992) Health women's way: Learning to listen. In: Koblinsky, M., Timyan, J., and Gay, J. (eds), *The Health of Women: A Global Perspective.*

Department of Statistics (1993) Personal communication, Prasuti Griha, Kathmandu.

Ehrenricht, B. and English, D. (1979) *For Her Own Good.* Anchor Books, New York.

Feuerstein, M. (1993) *Turning the Tide: Safe Motherhood, A District Action Manual.* The Macmillan Press, London.

Jeffery, R., Jeffery, P., and Lyon, A. (1984) Only cord cutters? Midwifery and childbirth in rural North India. *Social Action,* **34**(3): 229–250.

Levitt, M.J. (1988) *From Sickles to Scissors: Birth, Traditional Birth Attendants and Perinatal Health Development in Nepal.* Michigan University Dissertation Publications, Ann Arbour.

Levitt, M.J. (1993) *A Systematic Study of Birth and Traditional Birth Attendants in Nepal.* John Snow International, Nepal.

Maine, D. (1991) *Safe Motherhood Programs: Options and Issues.* Center for Population and Family Health, Columbia University, New York.

Maine, D. (1992) Cost-effectiveness of different safe motherhood programme options. *Safe Motherhood Supplement,* **9**(July–October). WHO, Geneva.

Manglay-Maglacas, A. (1990) Traditional birth attendants. In: Wallace, H.M. and Giri, K. (eds), *Health Care of Women and Children in Developing Countries.* Third Party Publishing Country, Oakland.

Maskey, B., Levitt, M., and Simpson-Herbert, M. (1991) *Maternal and Child Health: Management Issues at Community, Health Post and District Levels.* Division of Nursing, Ministry of Health of Nepal, Kathmandu.

Minden, M. (1993) Ke Garne? TBA training in Nepal. In: *Proceedings of the International Confederation of Midwives 23rd Congress,* Vancouver.

Minden, M. (1995) In whose interest? Women's experiences of hospital birth in Nepal. In: Murray, S. (ed.), *Baby Friendly/Mother Friendly, Vol. I, International Perspectives on Midwifery.* Mosby/Times Mirror International Publishers, London.

NORAD (1992) *The Logical Framework Approach (LFA).* Norwegian Agency for Development Cooperation, Oslo.

Pakistan Society of Physicians (1993), Eighth Annual Symposium. Nosocomial Infections. Reported in *National Health,* April–June.

Population Report (1980) **8,** 437–492. Johns Hopkins University, Baltimore.

Ransome-Kuti, O. (1992) Human Resources – a new breed of doctors. *NU,* **6**(1): 13–19.

Richards, M.P.M. (1978) A place of safety? An examination of the risks of hospital delivery. In: Kitzinger, S. and Davis, J. (eds), *The Place of Birth.* Oxford University Press, Oxford.

SWACH (1992) *Development, Use and Health Impact of Simple Delivery Kits in Selected Districts of India.* Report submitted to WHO, Geneva.

Tew, M. (1978) The case against hospital deliveries. In: Kitzinger, S. and Davis, J. (eds), *The Place of Birth.* Oxford University Press, Oxford.

Tew, M. (1990) *Safer Childbirth? A Critical History of Maternity Care.* Chapman & Hall, London.

Timyan, J., Brechin, G., Measham, D., and Ogunleye, B. (1992) Access to care: More than a problem of distance. In: Koblinsky, M., Timyan, J., and Gay, J. (eds), *The Health of Women: A Global Perspective.* Westview Press, Boulder.

UNICEF (1993) *The State Of The World's Children.* Oxford University Press, Oxford.

Walsh, J.A., Measham, A.R., Feifer, C.N., and Gertler, P.J. (1994) The impact of maternal health improvement on perinatal survival: Cost-effective alternatives. *International Journal of Health Planning and Management,* **9**(2): 131–149.

WHO (1991) What is the safe motherhood initiative? *Safe Motherhood Newsletter,* **4**:1.

WHO (1992a) Safe motherhood programmes: The essential elements. *Safe Motherhood Newsletter,* **9**, July–October.

WHO (1992b) *Traditional Birth Attendants.* A Joint WHO/UNICEF/UNFPA Statement, Geneva.

Wong, V.T. (1992) Introduction: Workshop on obstetric and maternity care. *International Journal of Obstetrics and Gynaecology,* **38**(Suppl): S3–S5.

Midwifery Education for the Future – The Needs of 'Developing' Countries

Gloria A. Betts

INTRODUCTION

There have been many initiatives taken in recent years to try to promote safe motherhood. However, maternal mortality does not seem to have decreased appreciably in those developing countries where the need is greatest. The reasons for this are manifold. Internal and border wars, economic crises, and structural adjustment programmes have all taken their toll. Nonetheless, we also have to ask ourselves what may be wrong with maternity service provision and midwifery professional education as they now stand. There is need for every Ministry of Health to make a radical reappraisal of the role that its midwives should be fulfilling in today's reality. In this chapter, the needs at different levels of maternity care are reconsidered, and some suggestions for an appropriate midwifery education for the future are made.

THE MIDWIFE'S ROLE AT VILLAGE OR COMMUNITY LEVEL

The professional midwife does not usually reside at village level, but she does have to train and supervise personnel who work with the community. Furthermore, she needs to be able to motivate communities to participate in the provision of services. This could include facilitating the building of health posts through community self-help, or working to ensure safe, available transport for the transfer of referred mothers through a system of household contributions.

In addition to sound basic midwifery skills, the midwife needs community development, communication and counselling, and training skills. She needs to be able to communicate effectively with different sectors of the community, from addressing the special problems of young people, in and out of school, to providing appropriate training and on-going supervision to traditional birth attendants (TBAs) and other carers in the non-formal sector. She needs to learn how to conduct surveys, and how to help communities determine and prioritize their needs through focus-group discussion and other assessment methods. She may find it useful to teach the Triple 'A' approach – Assessment, Analysis, Action – to help carers identify and solve problems.

Today's midwife needs to know about fund-raising if she is to help the women she serves. In this, the midwifery association and individual influential midwives may be able to give her back-up. They may liaise with agencies, non-government organizations (NGOs), and others who are interested in women's issues and provide income generation and business-skill training for rural women, to enhance women's financial independence. Women may have to be encouraged and helped to form their own local health insurance, so that they can have money to buy drugs and pay for services in emergencies, rather than depend on a welfare state that does not exist in practice, or on partners and relatives who are unable or unwilling to find funds for saving life, but manage to find funds for burial. In the western area of Sierra Leone, women had already created funds and insurance for their business activities, and were simply encouraged to expand on this for their health needs (Sierra Leone Midwives Association, 1993).

The midwife may also wish to aid the formation and training of Village Development Committees, or to help look for funds to establish low-interest revolving loan schemes. Village Health and/or Development Committees are important in promoting community participation. They can help bridge the gap between health-care providers and beneficiaries. Many have found the Bamako Initiative to be of advantage to their people. This initiative was launched by WHO and UNICEF in 1987 and involves a series of public health reforms. The package includes the establishment of cost-recovery systems for essential drugs. These can ensure the sustainability of drug supplies and improve quality of services, minimizing cost and allowing for the sharing of profits. In some projects, 10–50% of the profit is given to the community, to be spent on identified and agreed community development programmes (McPake, 1994). The midwife may be the professional in charge of the drug kit, but even if she is not, she has a role in informing the community about its availability, value, and benefits.

Unauthorized and uncontrolled fees for services can cause delay and sometimes maternal death, but there may be ways in which midwives can persuade clients and their families, interested groups, and philanthropists to support health centres in both kind and cash; thus, the upgrading of facilities and purchase of basic essential equipment can take place. Donors and NGOs could also be encouraged to adopt communities or districts and help provide infrastructure, supplies, and equipment (Betts, 1990).

THE ROLE OF THE MIDWIFE AT FIRST REFERRAL LEVEL
Various categories of personnel work at this level, but it is certainly advantageous to have a midwife at the community health-centre level. This midwife needs clinical skills for the prevention, early recognition, management, and emergency intervention of conditions related to the five major causes of maternal mortality (Betts, 1990; Maine, 1990; Kwast, 1991; Murray, 1993). Depending on the degree of isolation of the facility, she may need the skills for many or all of the following:

- Administration of intravenous infusion and other fluids appropriate for the replacement of blood loss.
- Emergency treatment for severe pre-eclampsia and eclampsia, including initiation of sedation.
- Use of the partograph for early detection of prolonged labour.

- Family planning services, prescription and administration of oral contraceptives, and insertion of intrauterine contraceptive devices (IUCDs).
- Emergency evacuation of retained products of conception.
- Manual removal of placenta.
- Initiation of antibiotics, both intramuscular and intravenous.
- Vacuum extraction, low forceps delivery, and emergency caesarean section.

Some obstetricians still jealously guard 'their' domain, but some countries have accepted that properly trained midwives can perform essential obstetric functions. A few have further tried and proved that selected midwives can be trained to perform emergency caesarean sections, repair ruptured uteri, and perform hysterectomies with the same success as physicians, thereby drastically reducing maternal deaths (Sanjiva, 1989; Duale, 1992).

In addition to the provision of good clinical midwifery services appropriate to practical needs, there is a need to use strategies that promote behavioural change. Midwives need to convince people that some traditional practices and beliefs are harmful. Using all the appropriate media, community elders, traditional leaders, religious leaders, and other influential groups have to be sensitized and motivated to help bring about any necessary changes in attitudes and practice in order to promote attendance at the antenatal clinic, the use of trained personnel for delivery, and the use of child immunization and modern family planning services.

The midwife requires management skills that will enable her to organize effectively her area of work, and control the resource materials, manpower, and money at her disposal. She needs to know how to make resources stretch, and what substitutes can be used when they do not. She should be able to develop standard protocols for the treatment of obstetric emergencies and other conditions that are prevalent in her area, and encourage service providers to use them. She needs to be able to collect health-related data, to have them analysed, and to use the results. This means understanding their meaning, sharing them with colleagues and policymakers, giving feedback to the relevant departments, communities, and other sectors, and planning the appropriate strategies to reduce mortality and morbidity. Skills are also needed in the fields of advocacy and lobbying (WHO, 1993).

The midwife has a unique potential role as a social change agent. She is very close to women and families and, if she is respected, she may act as a role model in many areas of public health, such as that of environmental hygiene. The importance of such informal education should not be underestimated. What families believe and how they behave can fundamentally influence their health and socioeconomic status, and can certainly affect the impact of the services that the midwife offers (ICM, 1987). The midwife needs to be a patient listener, who is willing to persevere and is determined to make progress with subtlety and without causing offence. Through focus-group discussions, midwives can find out what women think of the current service, what is acceptable, and what they would like or expect. In the light of the information acquired, interventions and practices can be modified to suit women's needs and comfort. The midwife is the professional person who is closest to the cultural and socioeconomic realities of families; she owes it to her clients and colleagues to pursue research in her practice.

THE MIDWIFE AT REGIONAL AND NATIONAL LEVEL

At this level the midwife is usually an experienced care provider, manager, or administrator in charge of units, she may be involved in policymaking and administration at ministerial level, or she may be working in, or be in-charge of, midwifery education institutions or programmes. To perform her duties efficiently, plan intelligently, and have the respect of health and other professionals with whom she has to interact, she needs to be educated at institutions of higher learning.

She needs the ability to examine critically the service delivery plans, and to be able to identify factors that adversely affect the profession. Policy design, implementation, and evaluation are all discussed and decided at this level. If midwives are not confident and assertive enough to advise, the consequences can be disastrous. As recommendations supported by research findings are more likely to be accepted and implemented, senior midwives must be fully competent in research awareness skills.

TODAY'S MIDWIFERY EDUCATION

Midwives need to be in control of their education and the policies that affect their practice. In many developing countries, the chairperson of the Midwives Board is still a doctor, and sometimes it is difficult to have desirable or necessary changes accepted, especially if the doctor perceives the changes as encroaching on the medical domain.

Presently, midwifery education in developing countries is didactic and teacher-centred, mainly a pouring in of knowledge. This is compounded by the lack of support materials, teaching aids, equipment, facilities, and human resources. The curriculum is often patterned on an out-dated model from a developed country. It neither meets the needs of the particular country, nor does it address the expanding role of the midwife in primary health care and social services. Today's education concentrates mainly on the clinical knowledge and skills required for antenatal care, management of labour, and the early postnatal period within facilities in which medical or obstetric back-up is fairly readily available. It rarely includes skills for the provision of essential obstetric functions so desperately needed in rural areas where the greater percentage of people live. Legislation, too, is out-dated in many countries and does not adequately protect midwives in their expanding practice (Kwast, 1991; Kwast and Bentley, 1991; Murray 1993).

Midwifery is taught mainly in hospitals where practice follows the medical model of client care, concentrating on doctors' directives; there is little concern for the socio-cultural aspects of care. In some areas, medical students, young doctors, and student midwives compete to attend deliveries and obstetricians vie for clients. There is not enough real experience in the community, where many of the obstetric emergencies occur.

National continuing education programmes are not organized on a regular basis and do not sufficiently make up for deficiencies in basic midwifery education. There are not enough programmes and the selection of participants is not always systematic (Betts, 1990).

There is a shortage of midwifery tutors in many developing countries. In part this is because many midwives are reluctant to pursue rigorous postgraduate studies when the conditions of service are not encouraging. It is also because national schools for higher midwifery education are few, and sponsorships to go abroad are not readily available. While nursing education and clinical practice have been enhanced in recent years, only lip service is being paid to midwifery education and practice.

MIDWIFERY EDUCATION FOR THE FUTURE

If the midwife is to function effectively, the education she receives must be structured as outlined above to give her the competencies and skills that she needs to improve the quality of life of mothers, babies, and families. Whether trained in or out of the country, the environment in which the midwife is going to work must be kept in focus when the educational programme is planned; situations can be simulated if necessary. If a midwife has to go to a developed country to train and therefore seldom have to cope with obstetric emergencies on her own, she will need additional practice in life-saving skills. Wherever possible, a student midwife should be helped to gain additional experience in communities that are similar to her own.

Wherever her education is conducted, be it hospital-based, community-based, or in a college of higher education, it needs to recognize the rapidly changing political and social climate and environment. The preparation should be one that enables the midwife to transfer knowledge and skills gained in one area to another area of work, and to be accomplished in problem-solving. The midwife of the future must be prepared to be competent and creative to cope with a lifetime of adaptation to new, complex, and ambiguous situations (Wringe, 1988; Burnard, 1990; WHO, 1993).

The curriculum must be one that will:

- Help the midwife to understand the various social, political, economic, and cultural influences on the environment and therefore the level of development and productivity. She should consider whether communities are being mobilized or encouraged to participate in health care provision, and be able to assess the status of the government's commitment.
- Make the midwife aware of the current epidemiological changes, health care policies, and available resources that will set the stage for her practice. She needs to be able to judge the need to lobby, advocate, or negotiate.
- Encourage the midwife to develop a positive attitude towards the community that she serves and towards other service providers. This will enable her to perform her roles and functions effectively, and empower her to cope both with inter-sectoral power struggles and with the cultural beliefs and practices of communities.
- Stimulate the midwife to acquire the knowledge and skills that will make her competent in performing her multipurpose responsibilities in caring for mothers, babies, and families. These should specifically include the life-saving skills that will enable her to carry out certain essential obstetric functions in rural settings.
- Help the midwife to grow professionally and encourage her to contribute to midwifery education at all levels, to share her experience through publications, newsletters, or magazines, and to conduct research into midwifery practice and the needs of the profession.

Women are becoming more aware of their rights and, before long, midwives will have to be equipped to handle moral, legal, and professional issues. They need to be concerned with ethical issues and to be accountable and responsible for promoting quality care and informed client choice in all areas of safe motherhood and child survival (ICM, 1993). Misuse of technology and excessive medicalization of care has to be guarded against.

Midwifery students could share a core curriculum with other health care providers, such as physiotherapists, radiographers, and laboratory technicians. These core subjects might include the social sciences, such as sociology, psychology, cross-cultural communication, counselling, logic, and ethics.

The cyclical approach of curriculum planning is useful; it focuses on the precise needs of the geographical area and produces a midwife whose services will meet those needs. The curriculum is designed after a needs assessment, which establishes the rationale for change, identifies key resources, and ensures that they are available. After this, the course content is organized and the learning experience, both teaching method and environment, is planned. A balance must be maintained between theory and practice, and care should be taken to ensure that practice is in hospital and community settings. Evaluation by student-completed questionnaires at the middle and end of training, and the use of periodic focus-group discussions with service users and target groups indicate whether the objectives are being met. The faculty can then determine if any restructuring should be done to make the educational process more relevant and effective.

TEACHING STYLES

Future midwifery education needs to be more andragogical in its approach and student-centred. Teachers need to be facilitators, and students should be encouraged to take responsibility for their learning. They have to learn to become questioning, reflective practitioners who are able to identify strengths and weaknesses in their learning and develop strategies to overcome such weaknesses (Burnard, 1990; Knowles, 1984; Winge, 1988).

Teaching methods should be innovative and stimulating; students have talents that could stay dormant if they are not stimulated to use them. In place of didactic methods, case studies – hypothetical or real, drama, role play, group work, discussion, and specific periods spent in the community – all help students to grasp the reality of a life situation. Where technology is available, students should be encouraged to produce their own home-made videos and slides, which could also be used to teach the community. Those who are artistic can help to produce posters and health messages in local languages. They can also learn to use drama to raise specific issues and to initiate the discussion necessary to solve a problem.

Students should be supported in their quest to acquire skills. This means that midwife managers of clinical areas must appreciate that a student's clinical experience period is primarily for learning according to the curriculum requirement, and not for providing an extra pair of hands to ease the burden of understaffed service areas. Managers must accept and be committed to their responsibility of helping students acquire the necessary competence. Tutorial and/or faculty members must continue to advocate to protect valuable student time and develop strategies to minimize conflict between institutions and clinical areas.

Where manpower and financial resources are limited, the location of schools of midwifery has to be considered carefully; such as whether there should be schools in each district or whether there should be a few well-equipped institutions in the country. Small schools are often ill-equipped, but sometimes when students are moved far away from their original culture and locality to areas with better social facilities, they are reluctant to return after completion of their studies.

DIRECT ENTRY INTO MIDWIFERY TRAINING

Direct entry into midwifery training has many supporters, because it is less disease-oriented and views pregnancy as normal rather than pathological. For this reason, the idea has recently gained in popularity in countries such as the UK. In developing countries, however, direct entry students have been accepted in the past at a lower basic general educational level than the post-basic students. Training was of a shorter duration and often did not adequately address the medical conditions that can complicate pregnancy. When this category of staff were posted to stations where both nursing and midwifery skills were needed, they were disadvantaged, because their scope of practice was limited. This training has therefore been phased out in many countries.

If direct entry is to be re-introduced, then the academic entry requirements must be the same as for the post-basic students. This will give students the necessary educational foundation to understand all the facets required to become an efficient midwife. They should not be trained as inferior practitioners, because this results in adverse personal and professional consequences.

CONTINUING EDUCATION

Continuing in-service education is crucial for midwives in developing countries, to keep them updated with rapidly changing information and procedures. Managers should have a plan which ensures rotation in attending such courses, so that the same people do not attend all the courses. There should also be provision for those who attend a course to multiply its effect by sharing the information gained with colleagues, thereby ensuring a larger number of beneficiaries.

Midwives in tutorial areas, senior management, and policymaking positions in developing countries definitely need the quality of education that will enable them to think critically, stimulate them to be innovative, and empower them to formulate appropriate policies as a result of research. Well-planned degree and Masters courses, with curricula based on the identified needs of a country, can give good preparation to senior midwives and help eradicate some of the set-backs caused by gender issues. Because midwifery is a female-dominated profession, midwives do not always receive the recognition that they deserve; preparation at this level not only enhances the status of the profession, but can also help to solve the problem of equities in salaries and rewards. This might especially be the case if there was a shared core curriculum with other health care professionals.

Distance learning or correspondence courses may be useful ways of enabling midwives in developing countries to further their education, but whose countries do not have the resources for the education they require, or whose family and other commitments do not allow them to undertake institutional studies.

Exchange programmes between practitioners from developing and developed countries can be of value to both parties – there is much to be learnt from each other.

CONCLUSION

The current basic midwifery education is not broad-based enough to prepare practitioners for the expanding roles and responsibilities required in the care for mothers, children, families, and communities. Midwives will have to be educated with the appropriate skills, knowledge, and attitudes to enable them to function as confident, autonomous practitioners according to the needs of their communities, and to make full use of the available resources (which should be evenly distributed). Pregnancy and childbirth need to be seen as normal physiological processes, rather than as conditions of pathological origin; but at the same time midwives need skills that will enable them to function effectively when problems arise, especially in areas where medical aid is not readily available. Midwives will have to strive continually for improved client care, to eliminate harmful practices, to protect against unnecessary interventions, and to ensure that technology and science are not misused. They may have to act as facilitators to families and communities, and also as co-ordinators for area-based community maternal and child health programmes.

There is no doubt that a good quality of education better prepares the midwife for her multipurpose roles and responsibilities. Well-educated midwives who can manage resources, negotiate, lobby, use modern management techniques, and advise policymakers confidently, using the results of research findings, will skilfully bring about the changes that are needed for the service delivery required in the twenty-first century. Thereby, they will make safe motherhood more of a reality in developing countries.

REFERENCES

Betts, G. (1990) *The Midwives Role in the Control of Maternal Mortality.* Paper presented on behalf of the International Confederation of Midwives (ICM) at the SOGON Safe Motherhood Conference, Abuja, Nigeria.

Burnard, P. (1990) *Students' Experience: Adult Learning and Mentorship Revisited.*

Duale, S. (1992) Delegation of responsibility in maternity care in Karawa rural health zone, Zaire. *International Journal of Gynaecology and Obstetrics,* **38**(Suppl.): 33–35.

ICM (1987) *Women's Health and the Midwife – A Global Perspective.* Report of a collaborative ICM/WHO/UNICEF pre-congress workshop held at The Hague, Netherlands.

ICM (1993) *International Code of Ethics for Midwives.* International Confederation of Midwives, London.

Knowles, M. (1984) *Andragogy in Action.* Jossey Bass, San Francisco.

Kwast, B.E. (1991) Safe motherhood: a challenge to midwifery practice, *World Health Forum,* **12**: 1–6.

Kwast, B.E. and Bentley, J. (1991) Introducing confident midwives: midwifery education – action for safe motherhood. *Midwifery,* **7**: 8–19.

Maine, D. (1990) *Safe Motherhood Programmes: Options and Issues.* Center for Population and Family Health, Colombia University, New York.

McPake, B. (1994) Initiative for change – paying for health care. *Health Action,* **9**(June–Aug): 7.

Murray, S.F. (1993) Appropriate training for midwives. *Nyatt om U-Landshalsovard,* **1**(7): 33–36.

Sanjiva, W. (1989) Taking up scalpel for babies in the breech. *Hospital Doctor,* **30**: 20.

Sierra Leone Midwives Association (1993) *Activity Report.* The 36th World Health Assembly Report, 12th plenary meeting, WHA 36.11.

WHO (1993) *Study Group Report on Nursing and Midwifery beyond the Year 2000.* WHO, Geneva.

Wringe, C. (1988) *Understanding Educational Aims.* Unwin Hyman, London.

CHAPTER

10

The MotherCare Project, Nigeria: A Step in a Revolution in Midwifery Education and Practice

Abimbola Olufunmilola Payne

BACKGROUND

During the past few years many of the international professional bodies have begun to discuss the midwife's 'extended role' and to recognize that new educational needs must be met if this role is to be fulfilled.

The pre-congress workshop of the International Confederation of Midwives (ICM/WHO/UNICEF, 1987), at The Hague, emphasized the need to review the midwife's role in women's health care. It argued that health providers must involve other professional sector organizations and governments to ensure that services reach the community. Three years later, in collaboration with the World Health Organization (WHO) and United Nations Children's Fund (UNICEF), the ICM held another pre-congress workshop in Kobe, Japan. At this workshop, which addressed the issue of education of the midwife, the message was clear that the midwife needed additional preparation to be able to deal competently and confidently with the problems and complications that lead to maternal mortality and morbidity.

The International Federation of Gynaecology and Obstetrics (FIGO) at its pre-congress workshop held in Singapore in September 1991, discussed the delegation of responsibilities to other maternal health care providers. The importance of an update in education and skills for the midwife to face the challenges of the new responsibilities, and to intervene in crises and complications, was also endorsed at the XIII World Congress of Obstetricians and Gynaecologists. A partnership between National Societies of Obstetricians and Gynaecologists and Midwives' and Nurses' Councils was recommended.

This chapter describes an in-service training project for midwives in Nigeria which combined training in life-saving skills with sessions in interpersonal communication and counselling skills.

NIGERIA'S PROFILE

Nigeria is rated as having the second highest maternal mortality rate in Africa (800–1500/100,000 live births). The 1990 *Nigeria Demographic and Health Survey* (NDHS) (Federal Office of Statistics, 1990) showed that only about 57% of women received antenatal care from professionals, 35% did not receive any antenatal care, and 4% received antenatal care from traditional birth attendants (TBAs). The majority of births were at home (60%). Mothers in high-risk categories, such as women less than 20 years old or who already had 6 or more children, were among those who delivered at home. Only 32% of these women delivered their babies with the assistance of a trained health worker. The NDHS also showed that the higher the level of education the more the woman avails herself of prenatal care.

The number of practising midwives in Nigeria was estimated to be 62,386 as of December 1993, for a population of approximately 18,585,000 women of child-bearing age (a ratio of 1/297). Midwifery education and practice in Nigeria is controlled by the Nursing and Midwifery Council of Nigeria. For comparison, the total number of doctors in Nigeria in 1993 was 12,466, a ratio of doctors to population of 1/7099. There is a maldistribution of health care providers, with a relative concentration in the urban areas and with more in the south than the north. In the northern state of Bauchi, for example, in 1993 the doctor/population ratio was 1:33,034, yet in Oyo state in the south, it was 1:3189.

Relationships between health care providers and clients have, for a long time, been unsatisfactory. Many midwives have been lethargic, uncommitted, and very passive in the execution of their maternal care services. They would explain this attitude as the end result of frustration, lack of incentives, and lack of infrastructure and tools with which to work. The attitude and relationship with their clientele and with community service providers, such as TBAs, were such that the professional midwives were feared. This situation, of course, negatively affected referral, consultation, and, ultimately, the utilization of health facilities. Pregnant women would only come to the health facility as a last resort and, in many cases, in a moribund condition.

The maternal health care infrastructure in Nigeria is relatively poor, including in the two states in which MotherCare became involved. Antenatal clinics, where available, are overcrowded and it takes a considerable length of time (5–7 h) before the examinations, etc., are completed. Most women do not have access to these clinics because of distance. Even when a health facility is nearby, a doctor or professional midwife may not be readily available. This has led to many babies being delivered by TBAs, trained or untrained. Family planning services are available, but women, either because of cultural or religious practices or because the decisions are made by others (mother, in-laws, husband), do not avail themselves of these services. The practice of early marriage still exists in some parts of Nigeria. It is estimated that up to 40% of women in local areas marry before age of 18 years. Abortion is not legalized in Nigeria, and so a woman who procures abortion does so at the risk of her life and is not only open to prosecution, but also to persecution by her friends, family, and in-laws.

In areas of the country where primary health-care intervention has gained ground, health centres are available, but of course have not been equipped with blood banks and other emergency facilities necessary to deal with obstetric complications. In the northern part of Nigeria, villages are scattered widely, whereas in the southern part villages seem relatively nearer to one another. In both cases, however, the roads are often bad and, in the rainy season, sometimes become inaccessible, making referral difficult.

In addressing the scenario described above the government of Nigeria requested MotherCare/John Snow Inc. (JSI) (funded by USAID) to give technical co-operation in maternal health; MotherCare commenced the maternal health project in February 1992. Some safe motherhood activities were already taking place in Nigeria, championed by the Society of Obstetricians and Gynaecologists of Nigeria (SOGON), the Inner Wheel Club of Apapa, Lagos, the Intra African Committee, and some Universities which received funding from donor agencies. The main thrust of these had been a campaign to increase awareness of the causes of maternal mortality, sensitizing people to the need to make pregnancy and childbirth safe, and in the development of protocols. The MotherCare project, with its training and education intervention components, was to add to and strengthen those ongoing safe motherhood activities.

PROJECT FEATURES

The long-term goal was to contribute to a reduction in maternal and neonatal mortality and morbidity in Nigeria. There were *three initial objectives*:

- To seek approval and commitment of the national and selected state governments, key political persons, and professionals for project strategies and interventions developed by MotherCare.
- To increase the awareness and prompt response of the community (women, families, community health workers, and traditional maternal care providers) to the problems and complications of pregnancy.
- To improve the quality of care of the mother and neonate through the upgrading of knowledge and skills of clinical midwives and TBAs to enable them to respond to obstetric emergencies and to enhance their interpersonal communication skills.

The project as a whole, therefore, comprised four inter-related and integrated parts; the training of midwives in life-saving skills (LSS) and other relevant maternity care, the provision of information, education, and communication (IEC) initiatives, the training of TBAs, and the initiation of a National Breastfeeding Policy.

It is the specific interventions designed to meet the third objective, "the upgrading of knowledge and skills of clinical midwives and TBAs", which are examined in this case study.

Needs assessment

One of the first steps taken, once it had been established that Nigeria/MotherCare/USAID were to collaborate in addressing the issue of maternal health, was to conduct a facility/institution needs assessment. The purpose of the needs assessment was to assist in selecting states to host the project, and then to select training sites within those states. For a state to be eligible for involvement in the project there had to be an existing interest and activity in the safe motherhood area, and several preventable obstetric problems had to have been identified. There had to be a functioning midwifery school, technical assistance from the State to the Local Government Authority had to be acceptable, and there needed to be support and commitment from the State Ministry of Health and the Health Management Board to the intervention programme, both during and, importantly, after the life of the MotherCare project. States which already enjoyed support from other organizations, such as UNFPA and UNICEF, had some advantage.

The sites for the midwife training were to be state hospitals with at least 4000 deliveries per year, to give adequate opportunity for clinical practice to the trainee. The clinical area had to be conducive to training, there had to be enough nurses and/or midwives available for training, and adequate quantities of drugs and other supplies.

In compliance with national policy, a decision was made to site one training centre in northern Nigeria and another in the south – thus paving the way for acceptability of the project. Having agreed in principle on this siting of the training centres, however, MotherCare ensured that the criteria set for selecting training sites, trainers, and midwives for LSS were complied with. MotherCare further sought endorsement and commitment to the project by encouraging policy meetings, which were held and funded by the National and State Ministries of Health. A *Memorandum of Understanding* was signed between MotherCare/JSI/USAID on the one hand and the Federal Ministry of Health and State Ministries of Health on the other. It spelt out the roles of the National and State Ministries, the Hospital Management Boards, and the institutions. A 2-day National Policy Meeting was held in June 1992, following which two National Advisory Committees (Technical and Policy) were set up to give guidance to project staff, as well as to influence key government and political personnel so as to establish and/or effect a change in policy as and when necessary.

The midwife training component

It was necessary to conduct a training needs assessment to establish the level of midwifery education and practice prevailing in the country in general and in the two selected states in particular. The assessment considered the available infrastructure, the state of existing equipment, drug stock, supplies, and instruments, and the clinical skills which the midwives already possessed and how frequently they used these (*Figure 10.1*).

Maternal mortality in the two states is due to the five established and known direct causes, with haemorrhage being highest on the list. Anaemia is strongly associated with maternal mortality and morbidity. The training needs assessment revealed that records were poorly kept and midwives had little or no skills of use in obstetric emergencies. Infrastructure was poor, most equipment was old, and some irreparable.

With these findings in mind, the LSS manual which had been developed by American College of Nurse-Midwives (Marshall and Buffington, 1991) was reviewed and it was decided to use this for both the Trainers' Workshop and training midwives.

	Trained to do		Do regularly	Do in an emergency
	Yes	No		
Start IV infusion				
Bimanually compress the uterus (crude)				
Suture (repair) episiotomies				
Suture (repair) cervical lacerations				
Suture (repair) vaginal lacerations				
Suture (repair) fourth degree lacerations				
Perform external versions				
Perform internal versions				
Perform vacuum extractions				
Perform speculum examinations				
Perform bimanual examinations				
Monitor labour progress/use partograph				
Perform controlled cord traction				
Perform adult cardiopulmonary resuscitation				
Perform infant cardiopulmonary resuscitation				
Perform rectal infusion				
Perform intraperitoneal infusion				
Perform pelvimetry				
Manually remove placenta				

Figure 10.1 Training needs assessment: clinical skills.

The training involved nine modules in life-saving skills and six sessions in interpersonal communication and counselling. The life-saving skills modules were:

1. Introduction to Maternal Mortality.
2. Antenatal Risk Assessment and Treatment.
3. Monitoring Labour Progress (including use of the partograph).
4. Episiotomies and Repair of Lacerations.
5. Prevention and Treatment of Haemorrhage.
6. Resuscitation.
7. Prevention and Management of Sepsis.
8. Hydration and Rehydration.
9. Vacuum Extraction.

The six sessions in interpersonal communication and counselling were:

1. Barriers, Motivators, and Enablers to Care.
2. Values Clarification.
3. Interpersonal Communication.
4. Counselling.
5. Problem Solving.
6. Introduction to Community Assessment and Outreach.

Site preparation

The aim of site preparation was to gear staff, systems, and environment towards the training activities. A total number of 122 midwives were given a 2-day preparatory course. The training was directed mainly towards acquisition of skills in the use of a partograph and the antenatal risk assessment forms, and participants were midwives of the antenatal, labour, and delivery rooms. All the midwives were observed closely for the eventual selection of candidates as trainers. Criteria for selection as a trainer were that a candidate should be:

- A midwife, nurse-midwife, or physician who is registered to practise in Nigeria.
- Employed by the training site and familiar with the geographic area.
- Experienced in antenatal and intrapartum care, with five or more years' experience.

The candidate should also have:

- The full support from the matron and supervisors to have the time needed to prepare, conduct, and evaluate the LSS training.
- A keen interest in addressing the problem of maternal mortality and morbidity in Nigeria, and a willingness to work creatively on solutions to the problem.
- A willingness to work shifts, including nights and weekends, while trainees are present.
- A willingness to move into the community with the trainees and in preparation to receive trainees.
- A willingness to travel to the work sites of trainees to evaluate their performance after training.
- A working knowledge of the health care system and ability to mobilize resources in a timely fashion to support the training.

At the end of the site preparation, ten prospective LSS trainers were selected for the Trainers' Workshop.

Training of trainers

MotherCare conducted a 3.5-week workshop for the trainers (five from each training site – Oyo and Bauchi states). The course involved 3 days devoted to communications skills, problem solving, and community assessment. The remainder was intensively orientated towards clinical labour and delivery care. Each prospective trainer worked for a minimum of ten (8 h) shifts, as well as attending classes and demonstrations.

The curriculum for the trainers included the full LSS modules, as well as an introduction to factors relevant to adult education, and the development of lesson plans and timetables for LSS training. Participants of the site preparation training, the trainers, and the first batch of LSS trainees had the enviable privilege of learning from experts and consultants from MotherCare (Dr Barbara Kwast) and the American College of Nurse-Midwives (Dr Margaret Marshall and Ms Gail Allison), and from local information, education, and communication experts who supported the team.

Training midwives in life-saving skills

LSS provide the midwife with the ability and competence to deal with obstetric emergencies. Midwives were selected for training from first referral centres, in groups of ten using the criteria set for the selection of midwives. They needed to be Registered Nurse Midwives with at least 3 years' clinical experience in labour and delivery, an adequate number of deliveries per month, and experience in working in all shifts.

They also had to be willing and available to initiate training at their own institutions. The training took 3 weeks, with the major part of the period being spent in labour and/or delivery rooms. The course content followed the lines already described under the training of trainers, except that it did not deal with teaching methods.

The midwives' exposure to these new skills has built up a high level of competence and confidence. It has brought out a display of innovation and initiative which hitherto had been dormant in midwives. As one trainer said, "Gone now are the days when we helplessly watch women die, because we were confined to comforting them rather than dealing actively with the complications."

One midwife described how learning to use the partograph in monitoring labour had not only helped in the early detection of deviation from normal labour, but had awakened in her a sense of foresight into the possible complications and, of course, a preparedness to deal with the complications. By the time a doctor is called to perform a caesarean section, she now had ready everything needed. Before the LSS training, she had relied heavily on the doctor's constant review and the famous 'last order' – "get her ready for theatre."

PROJECT MODIFICATIONS

The original targets for training had been clinical midwives. However, it became apparent as the programme evolved that it would be beneficial to all concerned if the physicians and matrons required to give both technical and administrative support were also given selective LSS and interpersonal communication skills training, and were offered an insight into their expected roles. This initiative proved to be of tremendous importance for sustaining the newly trained midwives' practice when they returned to their base. A 3-day course run by two experienced obstetrician–gynaecologists, an external consultant, and LSS trainers was attended by 40 physicians and 57 matrons. By the end of the course, the physicians and matrons had come to see themselves as part of the project. An unprecedented allegiance between them and the LSS trainers and midwives was established. The cohesion and co-operation was such that all the bureaucracy and red tape disappeared. Everyone focused on the woman and the appropriate care she ought to receive. Support for each other in the maternity care system was exceptionally strong.

The matrons are now very much committed to the availability of all necessary systems at all times so that women can receive timely attention as and when they require it. And as one doctor said, "I relax better now when I'm on call, because I have implicit confidence in the judgement of the midwives who are on duty. Their performance level is high and effective. I am only called in extreme difficulties and for complications which require high technical and/or surgical intervention, such as caesarean section."

By the end of the 19-month project the 81 midwives originally trained had returned to their different health centres and further trained a second generation of 256 midwives. The two tutors selected as trainers, in collaboration with colleagues, have trained 230 student midwives in antenatal risk assessment, the partograph, and the active management of the third stage of labour. The practice of antenatal risk assessment and use of the partograph in monitoring labour has now been institutionalized in the main training sites and sub-centres.

TBA TRAINING
Refresher courses were given to 42 TBAs in both states, and as one TBA aptly said, "Never has there been a co-operation of this magnitude between the professional midwives and the TBAs in the history of our practice." Another said "We are no longer afraid to refer and accompany our clientele to the health centres" and yet another, "Since MotherCare introduced its project to our state and the midwives in the referral centres now participate in our training, we feel free and undaunted to consult them for advice." MotherCare had ensured that those midwives to whom TBAs would be referring their clientele were members of the training team. This allowed plenty of interaction between the TBAs and the midwives during the course. A rapport gradually became established, especially when the interpersonal communication and counselling skills were taught. During the TBA training a visit was arranged to the antenatal labour and delivery rooms of the maternity units which would serve as their referral centres. There they were received and conducted around by the midwives with whom they would collaborate in the care of their clientele.

RECORD KEEPING REFORM
In order to address the inadequacies in reporting and collection of data, antenatal clinic registers of booking and attendance, and delivery and post-delivery registers were reviewed against antenatal risk assessment and partograph forms. A less complicated and easy-to-track register format and system was established.

MONITORING AND EVALUATION
Right from the onset of the MotherCare project, assessment, monitoring, and evaluation tools were developed, and a bench mark for level of performance established. Monitoring and evaluation continued throughout the project. Pre- and post-tests were conducted in the classroom, and acceptable levels of immediate post-training tests were judged as a score of 70% (82% midwives of Bauchi state and 80.5% of those in Oyo/Osun state scored 70% and above). However, because the programme was

competency based, the assessment of trainees' performance was an on-going process at clinical sessions through direct observations by trainers, completion of check-lists, and evaluation forms. Utilization of the antenatal risk assessment and partograph forms was assessed for correctness in their completion, inferences, and timely intervention.

As trainees returned to base and put their skills into practice, the National Project Co-ordinator and trainers paid periodic visits to the centres and/or units to further monitor performance, and give support and added training if and when necessary. Tools used for the monitoring visits were incident-report forms, and a support-visit check-list to assess the level of performance in client management and counselling. Again, the correct completion of antenatal risk assessment and partograph forms and timely and appropriate management were all assessed. The condition of equipment, proper maintenance of clients' records, drug and supplies availability, correct drug administration, and the practice of aseptic techniques were all examined during monitoring visits. As part of the monitoring and evaluation, in-depth interviews with hospital management staff (Chief Nursing Officers; Chief Matrons) were also conducted to discern replication of the LSS training, the effect of LSS on record keeping, and if there is any linkage established with the community in terms of follow-up and referral from the community. An inventory of all the instruments and equipment was taken during each support visit.

IMPACT ON THE WIDER PROFESSION

The multiplier effect of training further trainers meant that for every original LSS midwife trained in the courses, there were a further 2.76 trained on the job in Bauchi state and 2.87 in Oyo/Osun states. This has important financial benefits. The success of this MotherCare project also inspired the initiation of new activities which will further enrich the project, such as midwife interventions within the community and the establishment of a maternal mortality audit.

Prior to the introduction of the post-registration training in LSS and interpersonal communication and counselling, midwifery practice in Nigeria was limited to what was contained in the syllabus of the Nursing and Midwifery Council of Nigeria, the licensing body, and backed by Decree 89 of 1979. Practice beyond the stipulation of the decree would lead to prosecution, but through policy reform and the inclusion of the Chairman of the Council on the Policy/Technical Committees of the project, the importance and urgency that midwives have LSS became very clear. LSS training was therefore incorporated under Section 12 of the Nursing and Midwifery Decree, which states that, "In the performance of its duties under this Decree, the Council shall from time to time seek to improve methods employed in the basic and post-basic education of nurses and midwives, and for that purpose the Council may co-operate with recognized bodies interested in the preparation of experimental schemes for the basic and post-basic education of nurses and midwives." This is also the instrument we have used in introducing selected LSS training to student midwives in the schools of midwifery in the two states. At this point in time, the Nursing and Midwifery Council of Nigeria is discussing the possibility of introducing LSS training into the curricula of midwifery schools, pending the time when the national syllabus will be due for a comprehensive review.

LESSONS LEARNED

Soliciting endorsement and commitment to the project through meetings, and adherence to the signed Memorandum of Understanding not only created a good environment for the midwives to work in, but has brought out the best in them in terms of skills, level of performance, collaboration, co-operation, and initiatives.

It was necessary to modify the project as it evolved, to include not only clinical midwives, but also nurse-midwives and physicians in management positions. This exercise gained important support, enriched the project, and proved cost-effective. We believe it is essential to feel the 'vibration' surrounding a project, and to be prepared to adjust in ways that will be beneficial to all.

Finally, the inclusion in the training not only of technical life-saving skills, but also of techniques of communication and counselling proved very important. It is these combined skills that enable a midwife to provide good quality of care to the women she serves.

CONCLUSION

The introduction of LSS and interpersonal communication and counselling skills training for midwives in the states of Bauchi and Oyo/Osun in Nigeria has been an important step in revolutionizing midwifery education and practice. We on the project have enjoyed considerable co-operation from federal and state governments, and the relevant professional bodies, such as the Nursing and Midwifery Council of Nigeria and the Society of Obstetricians and Gynaecologists, which are represented on our technical and policy committees. We are confident that with these newly acquired skills and the high level of the midwives' performance, many more key organizations, private voluntary agencies, and non-governmental organizations will show commitment in sustaining the programme and thus contribute to the reduction of maternal and neonatal mortality and morbidity in Nigeria.

REFERENCES

Federal Office of Statistics (1990) *Nigeria Demographic and Health Survey.* Federal Office of Statistics, Lagos. Published in collaboration with IRD/Macro International Inc., Colombia, Maryland.

ICM/WHO/UNICEF (1987) *Pre-Congress Workshop.* ICM/WHO/UNICEF, The Hague.

Marshall, M.A. and Buffingtan S.T. (1991) *Life Saving Skills Manual for Midwives.* American College of Nurse-Midwives (ACNM), Washington.

CHAPTER

11

Rediscovering Midwifery as Artistry – The Role of Supervision

Marie-Claude Foster

Most managers within maternity services view 'supervision' as an integral part of their job, to ensure staff competence and effectiveness. This chapter examines how supervision can be used to ensure the continuing education of both midwives and traditional birth attendants (TBAs), and to develop a full range of midwifery skills. It looks at the application of professional knowledge to practice and at what contributes to making an effective midwife practitioner. In particular, it explores the roles of intuition and artistry. Finally, it considers the implications of this discussion for supervision within the formal health sector and in supervising TBAs.

INTRODUCTION

Formal institutionalized education and training converted midwifery in many countries from an important traditional occupation for women to the status of a publicly recognized profession. Training has also been identified as crucial for TBAs and, furthermore, it is argued that any such initial training must be followed up by ongoing supervision (Walt, 1986; WHO, 1992). In countries such as the UK, national workshops and consultations have begun to review the role of supervision in the context of professional midwives' changing roles and responsibilities (Duff, 1994). Such developments suggest that supervision may usefully merit some close examination, so initially the importance of continuous education is examined and then a working definition of supervision in the context of this chapter is provided.

WHY CONTINUOUS EDUCATION?

Initial training gives people the basic skills and knowledge required to carry out their task. However, this is never sufficient if we want competent workers, as there is always room for development. A useful model of the learning process views learning as a cyclical process (*Figure 11.1*; Clarkson, 1994).

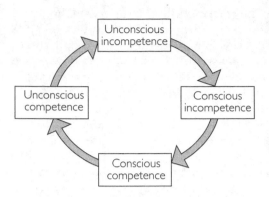

Figure 11.1 Learning as a cyclical process.

Unconscious incompetence refers to the stage at which we know so little about something that we simply do not know that we are incompetent. The next two phases are those of active learning. First, we become aware of our incompetence, an awareness that is crucial for learning to take place. And second, through what we learn we become consciously competent, this stage being a clumsy one in which we learn to put our new knowledge into practice. Finally, as we become more skilled we move into a stage of unconscious competence, in which we are highly proficient at what we are doing. If we remain static in this phase, however, sooner or later we become once again unconsciously incompetent as we fail to integrate changes which require new learning. Those readers who have learned to drive a car, for example, will be familiar with the process described. So, any practitioner who wishes to be effective needs to be continuously engaged in the learning process.

SUPERVISION – THE INSPECTION MODEL

'Supervision' is seen by some as a purely inspectorial activity, with the supervisor ensuring that the member of staff conforms to certain required standards. This is often carried out by the line manager. In this model of supervision, the supervisor is interested merely in checking that well-defined and clearly stated procedures are being carried out. This is a purely mechanistic strategy and the limitations of it are considered later, when what constitutes effective midwifery practice is discussed.

Inspection may also be accompanied by punitive sanctions for workers who transgress agreed policies. In some societies a dogmatic and punitive approach appears to be the norm in the workplace, especially in public sector organizations. But, it seems that at the personal level no individual wishes to be managed and supervised in this way. When the authoritarian, punitive style is used, it is often not so much a reflection of the wider society than an indication of the need and desire of the supervisor to treat others in a subordinate manner. For the (supposed) enhancement of their own status and prestige, supervisors and trainers may wilfully create role distance and exaggerate the existing hierarchical relationship between themselves and those they supervise. So, they may use the wider societal culture simply as an excuse for their actions. Supervision then becomes merely an act of control over workers and traditional midwives.

The inspection model may work in the short term, as long as supervisors are, at all times, in a position of scrutinizing the work of other midwives and that of TBAs through sheer coercion. But we know, from research in other types of organizations, that long term this style does not work and that sooner or later workers resist, often by sabotaging the efforts of project leaders and supervisors. Furthermore, it is actually impossible for any supervisor to keep a constant check over workers. To put it bluntly, when the supervisor is absent TBAs and midwives will do as they please. The inspection model is also unsuitable for supervision because it stifles the creativity of workers and they stop taking initiatives. As is demonstrated later, creativity is important to midwives and TBAs. For sustainability of programmes in which quality of service is valued, supervision needs to move away from the punitive–inspection model to one which supports and encourages workers to be self-motivated.

SUPERVISION FOR DEVELOPMENT

Supervision can be a quiet reflective time for workers to review both organizational and individual strengths and weaknesses in a supportive manner, where the accent is on learning and development. In this way, supervision could become a major medium for developing individuals, to inspire them and stimulate them to deliver a sensitive and high-quality service to mothers and their relatives. In many organizations nowadays, supervision refers to an educational activity, with the supervisor providing guidance and support as well as confronting and challenging the practitioner in an atmosphere conducive to learning. It is this educational definition of supervision which is considered here.

MIDWIFERY PRACTICE – A RATIONAL TECHNIQUE OR ARTISTRY?

As all professional midwives recognize, no amount of book learning adequately prepares for practice. Although book knowledge, guidelines, and procedures help, the competent practitioner is reacting all the time to the complexities she meets in the field. Standard training courses for both professional midwives and TBAs emphasize a technical rational model.

A technical rational model sees the practice of midwifery as a progression of distinct steps, processes, and procedures. From this perspective, there are definite 'right' and 'wrong' ways of doing things. And the application of this step-by-step guide ensures that correct decisions are taken. This model does allow for complexity in the real world, but generally complexity is broken into its parts and solutions applied to parts of the problems. The technical approach to medicine works from this model. For example, a midwife might consider the high blood pressure of a pregnant woman solely as a presenting symptom of a pathology in the course of a 'normal' pregnancy, and so use certain accepted medical interventions to reduce it, without seeing the need to take into account other issues in that woman's life.

Initial training and continuous education, including supervision, aim, in this model, to teach these technical, rational procedures to practitioners. The success of teaching here lies in the ability of the practitioner to apply these technical skills in a rational manner when she is in the field. The role of the supervisor becomes that of ensuring that these discrete skills are being applied in practice. From this perspective, supervision becomes checking that the known – theory – is being applied to the unknown – practice – and becomes simply a form of inspection (see Fish *et al.*, 1991, who discuss these models and have applied them to the supervision of student teachers and that of student health visitors).

However, there is a view that competent practice is not the application of technical, rational steps, but is in effect an 'artistry' (England, 1986). In 'practice as artistry' there are no set answers. The practitioner is informed by the knowledge gained from the rational–technical model, but her practice is holistic and comprehensive in approach. And in an unpredictable world, she draws on her intuition to create solutions.

I am not a midwife myself, but from listening to midwives, from my knowledge of what the job involves (Flint, 1986; Kitzinger, 1988) and, importantly, from my experience of motherhood, it seems to me that midwifery, when practised well, is indeed artistry. The technical–rational model offers solutions to precise, mechanistic, and objective issues in environments devoid of feelings. But this is not the world in which midwives and TBAs operate. Midwives deal with people at a highly sensitive phase in their lives, where the emotional, the psychological, and the subjective predominate. The medical model taught in midwifery is simply not appropriate to deal with this world. The techniques and procedures certainly help in saving and preserving life, but giving birth is much more than that. Thus, quality of service, for women and their families at that time, encompasses a strong relational element as well as the technical aspect. That relational element will always be, to a large extent, unpredictable. At times even the technical aspect of midwifery is unforeseeable. So, midwives have to be able to deal with uncertainty and the unknown. Rational models of decision making do not help when handling unpredictable events (Stacey, 1992). We need to draw on intuition to assist us in these circumstances (Agor, 1991).

INTUITION – WOMEN'S TRADITIONAL DECISION-MAKING PROCESS

Intuition, often described as a 'gut' feeling, tells us what to do especially when we do not know what to do and things are unclear and uncertain. It is through intuition that we arrive at a decision in unpredictable and complex situations.

It seems that intuition has been, throughout the ages, an important decision-making process. Women in their everyday lives are faced with very complex and unclear circumstances. Traditionally, it seems women have drawn on their intuition to guide them (Pinkola-Estes, 1993). In the Western world, with the rise of scientific rationality during the past 200 years, intuition as a means of decision-making has been much maligned. What has been given status and importance is the so-called rational step-by-step and precise form of decision-making. However, all this is now changing. In the field of management studies, psychologists and management researchers have discovered that the most important and useful means of decision-making in organizations is, in effect, intuition (see, e.g., Agor, 1991). What these writers tell us is that in running organizations – as in the practice of midwifery – people have to deal with unknown, uncertain, intricate, and perplexing situations, and top executives, especially the successful entrepreneurs of this world, draw on their intuition to guide them.

Work based on the theories of the psychologist Jung has drawn attention to the importance of intuition in contrast to thinking. 'Thinking' refers to a scientific-style analysis. Through thinking we compare and contrast, make deductions, and attempt to do so objectively by weighing the advantages and disadvantages of a decision.

Intuition is different in essence. It is holistic thought which sees how the parts fit into a whole – an important feature in midwifery if its practice is to move beyond a mechanical approach. Intuition tells us instinctively what we need to do next – often with us being unable to explain why we should take a certain course of action. It identifies patterns and, more importantly, the relationship between these patterns. The Jungian model also includes two other thought dimensions. Sensation is part of the thought process which draws on what is going on in actuality – it notices details. Feeling refers to taking note of emotions – joy, pain, grief, and fear. To be effective decision-makers we need to use all four dimensions – thinking, intuition, sensation, and feeling.

Here, we focus on intuition as it is quite often this thought-dimension which helps us decide the way forward when midwifery as artistry is being practised. Intuition is particularly useful when we are not sure of the correct course of action in uncertain and complex situations. When we do not know what to do, we experience discomfort, but if we acknowledge that we do not know and trust that our intuition will give us an answer, it appears inevitably to do so (see Henry, 1991, for a discussion of research in this field). Rational thinking in such a situation does not help much, but intuition will give us an insight. Some psychologists who have studied the learning process call it the 'Aha! experience', for when the insight comes we say "Ah! this is what I must do." However, rational thinking becomes useful *after* we have received our insight – when rational thinking helps us to decide whether this idea works in practice.

It seems that women are particularly good at using their intuition; certainly, this has been shown to be true for women managers (Agor, 1991). It is highly possible that TBAs also draw on their intuition to guide them. Unfortunately, the mechanical and technical training that professional midwives have received may have led them to under-use, or not to trust, their intuition. Supervisors need to be alerted to this. To inspire people to practise midwifery as artistry they have to encourage the use of intuition.

Intuition relies on 'gut' feelings and reflective thinking. If a supervisory session becomes a moment for quiet reflection, rather than a time for more didactic teaching, then the supervision process can foster the use of intuition. To stimulate intuition we need to move into a quiet space, which is relaxed and free from fear and anxiety. Fear is the greatest block to intuition. Supervision, it seems to me, is an ideal place to provide that type of environment.

ENCOURAGING REFLECTION-IN-PRACTICE – AN IMPORTANT ROLE FOR SUPERVISORS

Writing about professional knowledge and its application, Schön (1987, 1991) introduces the concept of the reflective practitioner by discussing the difference between reflection *on* action and reflection *in* action. In reflection on action, practitioners ponder after the event on issues arising from practical experience. This is, of course, an important component of supervision, where workers are encouraged to contemplate their actions in the field. But what is also required, and seems to differentiate excellent from inadequate practitioners, is reflection in action – that is, incessantly reflecting and finding appropriate interventions *during* practice. Here, the practitioner is aware that there is always a wide range of possible interventions, and it is the context that will dictate which one is appropriate. Although there may be preferable actions, there is not a rigid sense of a right way and a wrong way of doing things. The practitioner who constantly uses reflection-in-action does, indeed, draw on the guidance of rational, technical points, but this is not by itself sufficient. The practitioner is, at all times, creating and inventing solutions using her intuition – this is the essence of professional practice as artistry.

The analogy with the artist is a useful one. The artist does use techniques and procedures, but in such a creative manner that the outcome is in some sense always novel. The artist is not bound by technical issues. Too often, it seems, that in 'professional' midwifery training and supervision, the accent is on rigid techniques and procedures, which results in mothers and their relatives experiencing a dehumanized and inadequate service. For the creative midwifery practitioner, reflection in action is part and parcel of her work. Thought and action occur at the same time. The practitioner reflects on her knowledge and experiments on the spot. It is for the individual supervisor to discover what the situation is in her own environment. So, stimulating people to engage endlessly in reflection during practice is an important role for the enabling supervisor.

THE IMPORTANCE OF LEARNING

For supervisors who want to promote a creative approach to midwifery, it is not teaching which is important, but learning. Much work has been done over the years in the field of adult education, but it seems that these ideas have not necessarily reached professional training in the developing world. Teaching in a dogmatic hierarchical style seems to be the norm in the training of TBAs, and in many midwifery schools.

It is over 20 years since Rogers (1969) drew the attention of educators to the fact that it is only self-discovered learning which significantly influences behaviour. It follows from this that the supervisor is there to provide an environment which facilitates self-discovery for the student, with the latter being very active in the process of learning. This is very different from the expert model, in which the supervisor takes on a superior role and passes on expert knowledge to workers in a hierarchical manner. Education which liberates, as Freire (1972) argues, is not concerned with the mere transfer of information in a top-down manner. As empowerment is an important issue in the practice of midwifery, it is crucial that the atmosphere in which midwives and TBAs are supervised should be one which liberates and empowers.

Educationalists have distinguished between 'surface learning', in which people simply memorize facts, and the 'deep approach to learning', in which what matters is the meaning that the learner attaches to what is learnt. Drawing from this model, Gardiner (1989) looked at supervision in social work. He argues that adequate supervision requires attention to content – the 'what' of learning – and to process – the 'how' of learning. Further, and more importantly, effective supervisors are those who ensure that what Gardiner calls 'meta-learning' takes place. In meta-learning, there occurs the transfer of the content and process of learning from the original context, in which the learning takes place, to other situations where the context might be very different from the original one. The person who is being supervised becomes able to apply both content and process to varying circumstances in the field.

For supervision appropriate to promote meta-learning, the relationship between the supervisor and those she supervises needs to be appreciated. This relationship has to be an egalitarian one in which two-way learning occurs. It puts the supervisor in the humble role of learning from those she supervises – including 'uneducated' TBAs – and recognizing the significant and important knowledge that these people possess.

SUPERVISION AND MOTIVATION

Motivated workers are a valuable asset and supervision can be an important means to maintain motivation. People actually motivate themselves, so we cannot speak of supervisors motivating them, but the role for the supervisor is to create an environment where workers can be self-motivating. Many of the issues already discussed, such as style of supervision and emphasis on self-discovery in learning, are conducive to such an environment. Motivation is, of course, a very complex topic and there are wide individual differences, but we can say that motivation is an inter-relationship between the individual and the environment. Generally, it seems that people are intrinsically motivated to work well given the right circumstances.

Too often, it is the environment that acts as a demotivator. People need more than just to enjoy doing a good piece of work; they are social beings who need to feel that they belong to a social group. They also like to be in a position to exert some sort of influence and have some control over their work. The supervisor, therefore, needs to be aware that the social needs of 'belonging' are important for someone to work well, as are opportunities to exercise responsibility and to use discretion. An environment that is too constraining, for example, if workers are not allowed sufficient control over their work, needs to be changed to release people's potential, their energy, and their enthusiasm.

Supervisors may not be able personally to change whole systems, but they can make it known to their superiors that the organization itself may not be conducive to good work. Giving workers responsibilities and allowing them much use of their discretion are crucial to the artistry approach to midwifery. In a constraining system ruled by tight procedures and bureaucratic in style, any creativity is stifled and the worker is unable to engage in work as artistry.

SUPERVISION – A USEFUL MEDIUM FOR STAFF AND ORGANIZATIONAL DEVELOPMENT

The model of supervision as an educative and supportive relationship suggested here can be a very useful tool for developing both individual workers and the organization. 'Supervision as inspection' is not conducive to development. It alienates the individual, who often complies because she simply has to do so. And the wider organization misses out as it fails to learn from the wonderful pool of knowledge and expertise which 'ordinary' workers possess. It also misses out as it stifles the creativity and the capacity of workers to innovate.

It is the contact workers, that is the workers who are in direct contact with those they serve, who are the most important source of knowledge to the wider organization. Supervision of the kind suggested here can be a profound educational experience, from which the contact worker can derive much support. We know that people thrive from continuous development in which they use their talents to the full and expand their potential through continuous recycling of the learning process, discussed earlier in this chapter. Supervision can, therefore, be a central focus for the development of both individuals and the wider organization, development of the organization through it becoming a learning organization in which constant change (for deep learning is change) occurs.

IMPLICATIONS FOR PRACTISING SUPERVISORS

The major implications of this discussion are:

- Supervision is an important tool for developing and motivating staff. Continuous education is part and parcel of occupational development and all grades of staff need it –TBAs, midwives, and supervisors.
- For supervision to be an educative and supportive process, it needs to move away from an inspectorial–punitive model.
- Supervisors of midwives and TBAs require training in up-to-date educational methods that are appropriate for adult learners and lead to an environment in which people can feel empowered. It must not be assumed that midwives and/or supervisors 'know about education', because they are professionally trained. From what we know about the situation in the developing world, appropriate training of trainers and supervisors needs to be a top priority for any policymaker instituting TBAs' programmes or any other related projects.
- Supervisors and midwives have probably inherited a rational and technical approach to their work because of their professional training. Midwifery supervisors and trainers need to regain their intuition and creativity. They probably have much to learn from TBAs in this field and, when training and supervising TBAs, they have to guard against imposing a rational, technical model to midwifery.
- At a wider level, organizations which support these programmes need to embark upon a programme of organizational change and development. Too often, organizational structure and culture ensure that the innovative and creative skills of workers are stifled. To give good-quality service, the context in which workers operate needs to change to enable them to be given more discretion and responsibility in their work.

WHO SHOULD SUPERVISE?

It is sometimes suggested that supervision should be carried out by someone who is not the person's line manager. It is felt that this would make supportive rather than punitive supervision easier to provide. However, although line managers do have an auditing role, they should also have a role in developing staff and supporting them. In theory, therefore, line managers could also act as supervisors, but they would need training to be able to cope adequately with the inherent conflicting tensions in the double role.

Even when supervision is carried out by someone who is not a line manager, there are at times tensions in the role. Reviewing someone else's work, even at its best, has some elements of inspection. It is, therefore, particularly important when training supervisors to teach them to challenge and confront people in a supportive and non-judgemental manner so as to provide a positive learning experience for those they supervise.

POSSIBLE MODELS FOR SUPERVISION

The traditional model of supervision has a named supervisor working with an individual and spending time discussing and reflecting on aspects of the individual's work. At a practical level, individual supervision is expensive in terms of the time it takes and the logistics of meeting regularly, organizing transport, etc. Group supervision, where a number of midwives or TBAs are seen by the supervisor, is a good alternative. In this instance, the named supervisor needs to be thoroughly trained in understanding group dynamics and taught how to facilitate a group in a manner which empowers workers. In both models the supervisor has to guard against using a top-down authoritarian approach.

Other methods rely heavily on the peer group, that is, people working at the same level. Therefore, the peer group takes on the role of supervisor. Named people with special training, for example, in facilitating skills and human resources training may act in a facilitative role in setting up and supporting the peer group as and when required. Initially, these named people would have to teach the group about group dynamics and how to facilitate a group.

QUALITY AND CREATIVITY CIRCLES

Quality circles consist of people who do the same type of work and meet regularly, in official work time but on a voluntary basis, to discuss how to improve quality in the organization. Variants of this model can be used for supervision. The basic idea is that the group agrees to meet regularly and together look at how to improve quality of service and attempt to find creative and innovative solutions. In midwifery, as discussed earlier, quality of service comprises not only technical elements, but also, and more importantly, relational ones. Therefore, it is crucial to ensure that relational aspects of the interface between midwives and clients are considered.

ACTION LEARNING

Action learning is a process much used by managers, especially in the private sector. It was devised by Revans (1982), who discusses how in work there are 'puzzles' to which there are definite solutions. In midwifery these would be the purely technical aspects, where there is a known procedure or answer. However, in work situations, there are also 'problems' which are very complex and to which there are no ready-made solutions. These are the less tangible issues, of the type discussed earlier in the light of midwives dealing with the unpredictable and the uncertain. These particularly occur in the wider relational and emotional aspects of the midwife's work.

Action learning brings together small groups of people who work on real problems that they face in the field. So, it is firmly committed to dealing with very concrete situations. Together, people explore alternative solutions and the chosen solution is then tried out in practice. At a future meeting the workers report on successes and failures. Learning consists not only of looking at the problem but also of considering what the individual worker learns about herself. This is important if the solutions are to be transferred to other situations, as we all have patterns of behaving and acting which are not conducive to good work and which are often hidden from our own consciousness. An action-learning group, or 'set' as it is usually called, confronts and challenges these usual patterns. Group processes are important here also. The named supervisor would probably act as a group facilitator, encouraging an atmosphere in which both support and challenge are well balanced.

SELF AND PEER REVIEW

'Self and peer review' is a method in which the uneasiness of being confronted and challenged is made easier, because the person who is being supervised is in control of the process at all times. In small groups of four to six people, each individual's work is reviewed in turn. Time has to be allocated equally to each person, preferably with an hour, or an hour and a half, per person.

The group agrees on the area of performance or behaviour to be assessed. The individual selects criteria for reviewing and does her own self-assessment. She also controls the feedback she receives by setting what level of feedback she wants from the group. She can request that the group simply asks questions to help her clarify her thoughts, or that they make positive statements only. At a more challenging level, she can request negative feedback from colleagues, or even ask her peer group to act as 'devil's advocate' – that is to take on, for the sake of argument, the opposite view to the one which she takes.

Ground rules, i. e. the agreed basic ways of conduct in the group, are important here, as they are for the other methods discussed above. Useful ground rules are that everyone is committed to supporting each other, that self-disclosure and risk-taking are valued by the group, and that confidentiality is respected.

CONCLUSION

To conceive of supervision as a purely inspectorial activity is to miss out on tremendous opportunities. Supervision can become an important process in the continuous education and development of all grades of midwives and TBAs. Use of supervision for development with the sort of models outlined above can assist midwives to regain their artistry. It can enable them to give the sensitive service that all women are entitled to receive at that miraculous time in their lives when they give birth to a child.

REFERENCES

Agor, W. (1991) The logic of intuition – how top executives make decisions. In: Henry, J. (ed.), *Creative Management*. Sage Publications and Open University Press, London.

Clarkson, P. (1994) *The Achilles Syndrome: Overcoming the Secret Fear of Failure*. Element Books Ltd., Longmead, Shaftesbury, Dorset.

Duff, E. (1994) Meeting report: UKCC Working Conference on Supervision of Midwifery. *Midwives Chronicle and Nursing Notes*, November: 434–435.

England, H. (1986) *Social Work as Art: Making Sense for Good Practice*. Allen & Unwin, London.

Fish, D., Twinn, S., and Purr, B. (1991) *Promoting Reflection: Improving the Supervision of Practice in Health Visiting and Initial Teacher Training*. West London Institute of Higher Education, Twickenham.

Flint, C. (1986) *Sensitive Midwifery*. Heinemann, Oxford.

Freire, P. (1972) *Pedagogy of the Oppressed*. Penguin, Harmondsworth.

Gardiner, D.W.G. (1989) *The Anatomy of Supervision: Developing Learning and Professional Competence for Social Work Students*. Society for Research into Higher Education and Open University Press, Milton Keynes.

Henry, J. (ed.) (1991) *Creative Management*. Sage Publications and Open University Press, London.

Kitzinger, S. (ed.) (1988) *The Midwife Challenge*. Pandora Press, London.

Pinkola-Estes, C. (1993) *Women who Run with the Wolves.* Rider Publications, London.

Revans, R. (1983) *The ABC of Action Learning.* Chartwell Bratt, Bromley.

Rogers, C. (1969) *Freedom to learn: A View of what Education Might Become.* CE Merrill, Colombus, Ohio.

Schön, D. (1987) *Educating the Reflective Practitioner: Towards a New Design for Teaching and Learning in the Professions.* Jossey Bass, San Francisco.

Schön, D. (1991) *The Reflective Practitioner: How Professionals Think in Action.* Avebury, Aldershot.

Stacey, R. (1993) *Strategic Management and Organisational Dynamics.* Pitman Publishing, London.

Walt, G. (1986) Supervising trained traditional birth attendants. In: Mangay Maglacas, A. and Simons, J. (eds), *The Potential of the Traditional Birth Attendant.* WHO, Geneva.

WHO (1992) *Traditional Birth Attendants.* A Joint WHO/UNFPA/UNICEF Statement, WHO, Geneva.

CHAPTER

12

Organizing Midwives Internationally: The Story of the International Confederation of Midwives

Joan Walker and **Anne Thompson**

INTRODUCTION

Midwives from many countries have worked together for most of this century, crossing the boundaries of frontiers, cultures, and languages in order to improve standards of care for women and their babies. This chapter outlines the main features of that process as it unfolds through the work of the organization which the midwives set up – the International Confederation of Midwives (ICM). The major objective of the ICM is to provide a focus for exchange of midwifery knowledge in order to develop better standards of education for the profession and to strengthen its capacity to work for improved maternity and child health services in both developing and developed countries.

ICM's role has expanded as it has evolved. The account which follows describes ICM's structure, various modes of function, and different activities at national, regional, and international level. Today, ICM is a body of 68 midwifery organizations from more than 50 countries. In order to work effectively ICM has had to develop structures and strategies which offer the maximum level of participation to its member associations with the minimum level of central control. At the same time, world-wide mechanisms for specific, targeted intervention and representation of midwifery in major policymaking and decision-taking arenas have had to be established.

BRINGING MIDWIVES TOGETHER: THE BIRTH OF AN INTERNATIONAL ORGANIZATION

At the end of World War I, internationalism was in the air. People were sick of war and eager to reach out across national boundaries to others with similar interests and concerns. It was the time of the League of Nations, a time of idealism and hope. Into that world, in 1919, ICM, known then as the International Midwives Union (IMU), was born. Midwifery had neither the prestige of the established professions, such as law or medicine, nor the attraction of the new ones, such as radiography. There had been previous attempts to bring Europe's midwives together, and some of them, such as the Berlin Congress in 1900, had been very successful, drawing over 1000 participants from nine countries. Nonetheless, until 1919, no lasting structure had emerged and no permanent bond been created among the many midwifery organizations of Europe.

In the aftermath of that war, there was a growing public concern about the continuing high death rates among child-bearing women and their infants, which put maternal and child welfare high on the political agenda (Fildes *et al.*, 1992). In many respects, midwifery was a besieged profession during these inter-war years. The birth rate was dropping everywhere, doctors willing to care for child-bearing women were becoming both numerous and fashionable, and a number of other new-style health care professionals, such as health visitors and visiting nurses, were beginning to encroach on the community, the midwives' traditional practice base. In addition to this, more and more women across Europe were going into some form of maternity unit to have their babies. Midwives who delivered babies at home had to face radical changes in their working patterns, their education, and even their life-style if they were to survive as a distinct profession.

Although midwifery has a long history, it was, with few exceptions, without a formal structure at the beginning of this century. It continued to reflect the personal, intimate relationship which had formed the basis of the midwife's interaction with the women she cared for, mostly in their own homes (Marland, 1993).

Midwives were, on the whole, novices to the world of corporate action, particularly in the international field. The IMU was founded in the medieval city of Bruges in Belgium, and it seems symbolic that an organization which was eventually to represent midwifery organizations from every corner of the globe should start life in a small, crowded European country which had just been devastated by the worst war the world had ever seen.

IMU, the brain-child of a Belgian midwife, Marie Perneel, Matron of the Bruges Maternity Hospital, and Franz Daels, Professor of Obstetrics at the University of Ghent, set out to improve the services available to child-bearing women by campaigning for a stronger, better educated, and properly regulated midwifery profession. Public perception of the midwife was frequently coloured by the handywomen, or lay-midwives, who still practised extensively in Europe, particularly among the poor or in rural areas. While many nations, such as the Nordic countries and Germany, had implemented comprehensive state regulation on the practice of midwifery for many years, others offered little or nothing to the women who wished to establish themselves on a better professional and educational basis (Loudon, 1992).

CREATING AN INTERNATIONAL NETWORK

The initial move to unite a European grouping of midwifery organizations met with a swift and growing response. Starting with what was virtually a 'fringe' meeting of a handful of midwives from Belgium, Holland, and England, attached to multidisciplinary gatherings for nurses and social workers in Bruges and Antwerp, meetings of the IMU grew to over 1000 participants from 32 different countries within a few years. By the end of the 1930s full membership of the Confederation was held by Austria, Belgium, Bulgaria, Czechoslovakia, Poland, Denmark, England, Estonia, Finland, France, Germany, Italy, Latvia, Lithuania, Luxembourg, Sweden, Switzerland, and Yugoslavia.

During these early years, the organization hung together on the commitment and persistence of a handful of people. There was no fixed secretariat, and the Presidency rotated around Europe with the biennial meetings, which were hosted by the local midwifery association in membership with the IMU. Co-ordination and continuity were almost impossible to achieve under such circumstances and Professor Daels, who was the Secretary General up to the outbreak of World War II, worked tirelessly behind the scenes to hold the fragile network together and nurture its growth. He knew that effective communication was vital to the development of the organization. By 1932, a permanent record of congress proceedings, together with a report of IMU activities for the previous 2 years, was published in the journal *Communications*, in French, German, and English. This now remains a unique source of information about the IMU and the issues addressed by the midwives during the inter-war years.

The congresses of the 1920s show all the signs of a corporate body seeking its own distinct pattern of operation and clear identity. As with other women's organizations, IMU realized that the strength of an international body lay less with individual than with corporate membership. However, the organization took a number of years to clarify the most effective use of the biennial meetings, as there were complaints during the 1920s that host organizations were focusing more on matters of limited local interest than on issues commanding international concern. Despite these difficulties, and backed only by slender resources, the new international organization for midwives grew steadily.

PROFESSIONALIZING MIDWIFERY

By the 1930s there was a new, more assured note in the IMU's proceedings. The record of the 1934 Congress, held in London, stated that:

> *The International Federation of Midwives (sic) has for its object the protection of the mother and child. With this object in view the efforts and activities of the Federation shall at the same time be directed towards the scientific, moral, social, and economic improvement of the profession of midwife. (Communications, 1936)*

Each congress had a clear theme and there was vigorous debate around issues of midwifery education (in London, 1934), the place of birth (in Berlin, 1936), and the midwife's role as a social worker (in Paris, 1938). The country-by-country reports, published in *Communications* provide a fascinating overview of the development of the midwifery services throughout Europe during the inter-war decades. Sadly, the record is limited mainly to the published proceedings of the congresses, since the IMU's archives were lost in Ghent during World War II. Despite recurrent worries about funding and staffing, midwives now had a permanent international organization to represent them and to act as a forum for exchanging information and ideas on changes in practice, as well as to campaign for improved conditions throughout the maternity services.

One of the issues on which midwives in Europe took a vigorous and united stand was professional education. They recognized that high educational standards held the key to improved status and public recognition. There was a steady attempt to persuade the governments of European countries to introduce a 3-year minimum education programme for midwives. Some of the debates in congress have a very contemporary ring, with direct entry and the place of birth featuring regularly. More than 60 years later, midwives are once again focusing on these issues, worried about what is perceived by many to be a dehumanization of birth through undue routine intervention, as well as about the dilution of midwifery knowledge and skills through inadequate or inappropriate education programmes.

STARTING AGAIN

On the eve of World War II, in Paris, the IMU stepped beyond its usual, professional preoccupations to issue an impassioned plea for peace (*Communications*, 1939). This was the last that was to be heard of the IMU for more than 10 years. In 1954, after several years of tentative discussion and meetings in Rome and Paris, as well as in London, the decision was finally taken to relaunch the organization as the International Confederation of Midwives, with a permanent Secretariat based in London and a new constitution. Madame Mossé, the pre-war President, had long cherished the dream of an ICM reborn in France, and had even made provision in her will for premises for the Secretariat. However, her death in 1949 left the project without its strongest champion and the Royal College of Midwives in London set about the task of organizing the first full-scale congress since before World War II.

More than 50 countries sent representatives to the 1954 Congress, the first to see expansion of ICM membership well beyond the bounds of Europe. Little time was lost in putting the reorganized ICM on to the international political scene. By the end of the 1960s the ICM had held its congress outside Europe for the first time, in Chile, and 3 years later the congress went to the United States, where midwifery had been all but obliterated during the course of the century (Litoff, 1986).

BRINGING MIDWIFERY INTO THE UNITED NATIONS SYSTEM

As early as 1925 midwives in the IMU had campaigned for recognition by the League of Nations, in an effort to gain credibility as a professional body with international significance and to break the parochial stereotype from which midwives sometimes suffered. In the early 1960s the ICM was formally recognized as a non-governmental organization (NGO) accredited to the UN. This meant that the ICM had the right to send midwife delegates as official observers to all relevant UN agency meetings and that the ICM was acknowledged as the forum for consultation when the midwife's view on the health care of the mother and child was needed. Close collaborative links were rapidly established with agencies such as the World Health Organization (WHO), the United Nations Children's Fund (UNICEF), and the International Labour Office (ILO). An early consequence of this activity was the first draft of what was to become universally known as the *International Definition of the Midwife* (ICM/WHO/FIGO, 1990, 1992), a statement which was to be used as an international yardstick to establish the parameters of a midwife's practice and to help governments draft appropriate legislation for the profession (WHO Expert Committee, 1966).

MIDWIVES AND MEDICAL MEN

Professional rivalries between medical practitioners and midwives have been well-documented and seem to have been almost universal during the past two centuries, as competition for the right to care for child-bearing women and their families became more acute (Gélis, 1988; Donnison, 1989). In the face of this, the ICM set out to build bridges with those colleagues whom they acknowledged as vital partners in the effort to provide good-quality health care. Obstetricians, represented by the International Federation of Obstetricians and Gynaecologists (FIGO), and paediatricians, through the International Paediatric Association (IPA), recognized the value of such a partnership and helped create effective mechanisms for international NGOs concerned with reproductive and child health care to work with WHO and UNICEF.

One early result of this collaborative effort was the publication of *Maternity Care in the World, an International Survey of Midwifery Practice and Training*, a joint venture with FIGO, which surveyed the provision of maternity and family planning services in some 210 countries. Two editions were published, in 1966 and 1976, and provided a precious resource for policymakers and funding agencies (FIGO/ICM, 1966, 1976). As Dr Hafdan Mahler, then Director-General of WHO, said in his Foreword to the second edition, the report stressed the expanded role and functions of the professional midwife as a teacher and as a family counsellor. It also drew attention to the enormous disparities in reproductive health care provision between the industrialized countries and the less developed parts of the world, where up to 80% of women remained without any form of professional care throughout pregnancy and delivery.

These were the years where governments world-wide were struggling to establish health-care systems capable of offering a minimum service to everyone. During the early years of post-war economic recovery, there was a growing concern about the rapid increase in the world's population and the equitable distribution of finite resources. Developments in technology and pharmacology had made fertility control, at least in theory, realizable, and in many parts of the world social attitudes were changing quite rapidly.

As a result of these changes, and as an outcome of its earlier collaboration with FIGO, ICM began a massive programme on behalf of the United States Agency for International Development (USAID), conducting educational projects with midwives in family planning and in the training of traditional birth attendants (TBAs). Between 1972 and 1979, ICM held 20 inter-regional working parties involving more than 80 countries. Participants included obstetricians, family planning associations, government officials, and international agency representatives, as well as midwives. Generous funding from USAID had allowed ICM not only to take on the necessary staff to administer such a vast project, but also to become sufficiently established to move to its own premises. ICM's name became well-known via the complex outreach achieved through the USAID project, although it is worth noting that membership numbers did not increase greatly during this time.

REORGANIZATION

The burst of activity in relation to family planning and the training of TBAs could not last forever. Once USAID funding ceased at the end of the 1970s, ICM was thrown back on its own slender financial and professional resources. A period of anxious debate took place about whether and how the ICM could be re-established on a sustainable footing.

In 1981 a new constitution was voted by Council, and ICM once more began to play a significant role in international affairs concerned with child-bearing women and their babies, and with the education and regulation of the profession of midwifery. A process of regionalization, introduced through the new constitution, resulted in non-European members taking a more visibly active part in determining ICM's future direction.

The first ICM congress after this reorganization, in Australia in 1984, gave new vigour to many of the debates which have persisted throughout its history – the role and status of the midwife and the place of birth. Established once more on a small, but reasonably solid basis, the organization, which now numbered midwives from all over the world and from a wide range of cultures, was able to look in greater depth at the problems facing child-bearing women in the late twentieth century.

MIDWIVES MAKING MOTHERHOOD SAFER

In 1987, the world was made aware of the scandal of the death in childbirth of more than half a million women a year, 99% of which occurred in developing countries. The launch of the global Safe Motherhood Initiative (SMI), which highlighted this scandal at the WHO conference in Nairobi, Kenya, provided a focus for ICM's new energies (Kwast, 1991). Within months, ICM took up the challenge of maternal mortality at its 21st International Congress in The Hague, with the first of a series of collaborative Pre-Congress Workshops conducted in partnership with WHO and UNICEF.

At the Nairobi conference, WHO announced the target of reducing maternal deaths by 50% by the year 2000 (Mahler, 1987). The SMI provided a stimulus for women and midwives from all sorts of backgrounds to work together in many different ways to improve conditions of childbirth. Over the next 6 years, ICM undertook a systematic exploration of the main areas in which midwifery could make an effective contribution to SMI.

CHANGING PRACTICE

The first Pre-Congress Workshop, held in The Hague in 1987, brought together 44 participants from the 29 countries where maternal mortality rates were highest. It was designed to commit midwives to collective action and to ensure that all midwives became aware of the dimensions of the problem. The workshop focused on midwives' contribution to the social, economic, political, educational, and managerial factors directly impinging on maternal death and morbidity. The action statement issued by the participants at the close of the workshop contained a series of key strategies related to improvements in midwives' education, the full exercise of their life-saving skills, the development of resource management, and the prioritization of services and involvement in basic operational research (ICM/WHO/UNICEF, 1987).

Subsequent to this Pre-Congress Workshop, and in recognition that midwives are rarely prepared or properly placed to take up the role demanded of them by the SMI, follow-up activities were undertaken in many parts of the world. From the headquarters of ICM, two workshops were organized, supported by governments of the host country. The first, held in Accra, Ghana, in January 1989 (ICM, 1989), brought together 25 participants from five anglophone African countries and called upon them to produce national implementation plans to introduce feasible changes within the constraints of their existing health services and country situation. The second workshop, which re-iterated the theme of the first, took place a year later in Ouagodougou, Burkina Faso, with 42 participants from eight francophone countries (ICM, 1990).

Written reports from the participants 2 years after the Ghana Workshop showed that four major issues were commonly identified. First, there were insufficient professionally trained midwives as well as an uneven distribution of those who were trained. Second, there were not enough trainers or training. Third, there were poor antenatal services. Finally, particularly in rural areas, there were poor referral systems and processes.

The reports showed that change, in line with the original action plan, was ineffective as a result of lack of support from the national governments, of funding and resources, and of commitment of those involved. Positive action included the enactment of legislation, improvement of training, recruitment drives, the setting up of health centres, the building of river and horse-and-cart ambulances, increasing supplies of essential medicines and equipment, improving attendance rates at clinics or number of home visits during the antenatal and postnatal periods, and instigating family planning training and services (ICM, 1992a).

With the exception of two countries, assessors visited participants of the Burkina Faso workshop in their own countries 2 years after the event. Similar problems were encountered by the assessors as those identified in participants' reports. However, successes were noted, although the route of achievement was not always that originally planned. In one case the plan had not been launched, but the midwives who had participated in the workshop had formed an association and had looked for ways to set up post-basic education courses. In addition, they had submitted a proposal to their government designed to reduce the number of abortions among students through sex education in schools (ICM, 1992b).

Participants from another country realized that their particular plan was far too ambitious and had therefore abandoned all ideas of change, although their government had taken the initiative of printing partographs for midwives to use. Disillusionment and a lack of motivation, supervision, infrastructure, and organization were all contributing factors. The absence of co-operation, resources, and financial support had, sadly, outweighed the good intentions of almost all of the participants. They had returned to their countries fired with enthusiasm to effect change, bring about local initiatives, and determined to form and develop midwifery associations. Their achievements, although commendable in international and national eyes, were disappointing to the participants themselves, as they had envisaged greater collaboration and co-operation than had been achieved.

The relative isolation and lack of support experienced by many of the workshop participants on return to their own countries has not only endorsed the importance of ongoing support and follow-up, but has highlighted the importance of providing initial information to governments and ensuring adequate preparation of the person nominated to attend the workshops. As a follow-up measure, external evaluations of the implementation of workshop action plans designed by individual participants confer formal recognition of their efforts.

ADAPTING EDUCATION

Three years after The Hague Pre-Congress Workshop, a further workshop was held prior to the 22nd International Congress, in Kobe, Japan, in 1990. It was recognized that much of the education traditionally received by midwives in many countries failed to address the harsh clinical realities of the causes of maternal mortality and to provide the skills needed by midwives to combat the threat of maternal mortality. Furthermore, the education did not contextualize learning in the many varied settings in which midwives were called upon to practise. The focus of this workshop was to direct attention to ways in which midwives might be prepared, through education, to be confident and competent to cope with the realities of practice and meet the needs of child-bearing women, particularly in the community. The 35 participants examined the five major causes of maternal mortality and used these as a framework for a new, community-based approach to the midwifery curriculum. The four elements of community context, prevention, treatment, and follow-up were used to develop understanding and skills in the management of postpartum haemorrhage, obstructed labour, eclampsia, puerperal sepsis, and abortion.

The action statement issued at the close of this workshop stressed, among other things, the power of improved midwifery education programmes to affect the Safe Motherhood goals; the need for midwifery education to be recognized as being separate from that of nurse education; and the ability of the practising midwife to evaluate her own practice, especially in relation to the needs of the local community (ICM/WHO/UNICEF, 1990).

The enthusiasm generated by the workshop stimulated follow-up activities by midwifery associations in both developing and developed countries. The midwife participant from Tanzania set up a seminar for midwife educators and managers. This was the beginning of a lengthy process by which the whole education system for midwives was adapted to make it suitable for the needs of the women and families who use and benefit from the service.

Other activities in African countries included the recognition of major health problems in Ethiopia and a change to community-based education for midwives; collaboration between the American College of Nurse-Midwives, the Ministry of Health, and the Ghana Registered Midwives' Association in carrying out a project to train midwives in life-saving skills; workshops in Nigeria to enhance the training of midwives; and the development of pictorial cards for use by TBAs in Sierra Leone, improving record keeping and introducing use of the partograph by midwives.

Indonesia had an ambitious plan to train over 60,000 midwives. There were also plans to train midwife teachers, review the regulation controlling midwifery practice, and prepare literature for maternal and child health guidance in communities. Sri Lanka formulated demands to revise completely their education curriculum, including evening classes in English to enhance the overall knowledge base of the students.

In the developed world, meetings were held to scrutinize programmes and to ensure that Safe Motherhood was being promoted. For example, the midwives of Japan worked closely with two of their midwife associations to obtain a review of professional and continuing education for midwives and the development of a child health care network; also, by working with the Ministry of Health, a maternal health notebook was revised.

In Europe, too, midwives were taking the Safe Motherhood challenge seriously. The midwives of Germany concentrated their efforts in assisting their colleagues from the former East Germany by holding three workshops for them. They also financially supported a midwife from Sierra Leone to undertake training as a midwife tutor in Ghana.

The Royal College of Midwives, UK, concentrated their efforts on fund-raising on the first International Day of the Midwife on 5th May 1991. With the money raised they purchased equipment for midwives in Sierra Leone, Uganda, the former Soviet Union, and other countries. They also hosted midwives from other countries who visited the UK and have enabled midwives to act in the capacity of consultants in developing education curricula, particularly in Tanzania and Botswana.

COLLABORATION FOR SAFE MOTHERHOOD

In addition to ICM member-association activities, there have been regional activities, the largest event in recent years being a conference hosted by the Australian College of Midwives Incorporated. This attracted midwives from 17 countries in the Asia–Pacific region, a part of the world where communication and continuing education programmes for midwives are notoriously difficult to organize, across thousands of scattered islands. The papers presented provided insight into the variety and extent of the work of the midwife in the region.

A Pre-Conference Workshop based on the Kobe report developed an action statement by the 13 countries represented. It was recommended that strategies identified in the 'Framework for Implementation' devised by the workshop participants should be adopted within the maternal and child health services of the Asia–Pacific region. The framework addressed wide-ranging issues, including inequality for women, inaccessible and inadequate health care services, unregulated fertility, inadequacies of antenatal and postnatal care, lack of trained midwives, and inappropriate or inadequate midwifery education (Australian College of Midwives Incorporated, 1992).

Within Europe, the midwives in Germany hold regional conferences on a yearly basis. These are well-supported and documentation for those unable to attend is presented in the regular magazine produced by the Midwives' Association.

The value of the Pre-Congress Workshop reports was recognized, and spread far beyond member associations. Other international agencies have participated in workshops related to midwifery education, such as two held within the East Mediterranean region of WHO on the 'Elimination of Neonatal Tetanus', and have given encouragement to improve midwifery practice and training. UNICEF, for example, is giving institutional support within the State of Rajasthan, India, to the safe motherhood component, as well as preparing a booklet for field-level workers and promoting a 'Village Contact Action Drive on Safe Motherhood', an innovative approach in interpersonal communication.

The 'Kobe' framework has also provided the basis for community-based educational modules which have been developed by WHO and will soon be ready for use in many countries. These incorporate the principles of flexible, adaptable, and practical education for safe practice (Maclean and Tickner, 1992).

Individual countries have shown interest in various ways, as in the example of West China where a programme to initiate maternal and child health care, mainly through the training of village and township doctors and the provision of postpartum haemorrhage educational material for TBAs, is in progress.

QUALITY CARE FOR SAFER MOTHERHOOD

Adequate, functioning equipment and well-trained staff are only part of the equation which makes up an effective health-care system. There is growing evidence from around the world that many women fail to take up the maternity services available to them because they find them unacceptable. Staff attitudes are an important element in delivering an effective service, and are a vital part of quality care. Many midwives have not been taught how to monitor and evaluate the service they offer, and yet these skills are central to the adequacy and effectiveness of the service they provide.

The third Pre-Congress Workshop of the series, held in Vancouver, British Columbia, in May 1993, therefore worked on developing indicators for measuring the quality of care delivered. The 39 participants, representing 22 countries, worked in both the main group and in small group sessions, using material from the previous two Pre-Congress Workshops and material specially prepared for this workshop. The participants determined the constituents of quality midwifery care, and then evaluated current practice and developed new ways of monitoring and evaluation.

An action statement, which was not only distributed to participants of the workshop, but also to delegates attending the congress, clearly spelled out the roles of governments, international and professional agencies, and midwives (ICM/WHO/UNICEF, 1994). Each midwife also prepared an action plan for herself to implement on her return home.

Looking at what these midwives have achieved, it is clear that the commitment needs to be one of long, steady application to bring about beneficial change. In Zimbabwe, a counselling service for teenage mothers has been incorporated within the normal midwifery services, and a discussion group for midwives has been formed to address midwifery and research issues. Participants from Papua New Guinea tried to organize a midwifery group within the existing nursing association. The intention of the group was to share experience, ideas, and knowledge to benefit mothers and infants. Working with and through the Ethiopian Midwives' Association, the Ethiopian participant identified changes required in their education curriculum, as well as the need to update midwives on a regular basis. To effect this, workshops and refresher courses have been planned. A bonus to these midwives is the opening of a further midwifery training school in their country with plans for another school to be opened.

Implementing change, however much this is needed, is rarely easy, as the participants from Uganda discovered. Midwives need to create awareness among women and have organized instruction in women's homes, in clinics, and in hospitals. Some midwives required refresher courses, which have been adapted to incorporate life-saving skills and basic training on the use of partographs. A longer-term problem is the shortage of trained midwives in Uganda. Only about 150 are trained each year by the government and a few others by private institutions. Although TBAs have received training, it is difficult to follow-up their practice due to the high transport costs. Cultural beliefs and the negative attitudes of men are cited as a hindrance to the use of family planning across the board, but three centres have demonstrated that this can be safe, culturally acceptable, and effective.

Midwives in Cambodia recognized lack of knowledge, as a result of poor communication systems, to be a problem and have now formed a midwifery group which aims to share and disseminate information across the country. The absence of financial support and trained facilitators complicates their endeavours. A further complication is that information reaching Cambodia and many other developing countries is frequently in English, so needs to be translated into the local language. A 'cascade' approach is being tried; so far the midwives who attended the Pre-Congress Workshop have held five workshops for other midwives around the country. The strategy employed has been to use different facilitators on each workshop as a training exercise so that they can undertake their own workshops in the future (ICM/WHO/UNICEF, 1994).

One outcome of the three Pre-Congress Workshops is that midwives are assuming responsibility for recognizing and addressing the needs of women, babies, and families within their respective countries. In the developing countries from which the participants in the Pre-Congress Workshops have come, resources in human terms, as well as financial and logistic ones, are often scanty. It is to the midwives' credit that they are able to attend, share, develop plans, and then gradually effect change, often against all odds. Many of these countries suffer from famine, drought, civil unrest, war, earthquakes, or other disasters. Global problems, such as an inadequate safe water supply, no transport, or lack of health care facilities and personnel, are well-documented, and it is in these scenarios that the Pre-Congress Workshop participants are striving and slowly succeeding.

MEMBER ASSOCIATIONS

Since its inception in 1919, one of the hardest tasks that has persistently faced the ICM has been to help establish national, professional midwifery organizations. In most countries the organizations have emerged only after the profession has been legally regulated, although, as in a number of the newer organizations in the Canadian Provinces, they are occasionally formed to act as campaigning groups to lobby for the legal recognition of the profession.

In some countries the position of women in society still makes it difficult for midwives to organize themselves into a formal professional body. In today's society the literal meaning of the English word 'midwife' (with woman) is in evidence, as midwives around the world have sought to work and liaise with women's groups in campaigning for women's rights. The outcome of some of these enterprises includes changes in legislation to improve the hours and conditions of work for women, permitting or improving maternity leave, making provision for breastfeeding in places of work or in public places, and giving the woman a choice in the place of birth for her child and in her carer.

From its earliest days, ICM has seen the need to strengthen midwifery by nurturing associations as they develop, and in more recent years a special fund has been reserved for newer, smaller groups to join ICM. Just as it is recognized that midwives working with women's groups are able to achieve more than either group working independently, so it is recognized that midwives working together are able to pool their knowledge, learn from each other's experiences, and stand a better chance of being listened to. It is the collective voice which has been heard by politicians when the matter of legislation is considered and when agreement needs to be reached over standards for entry into midwifery training, or for recognition as a practising midwife. The international agencies are also more likely to work with an established midwifery association than with an individual midwife.

Most of the member associations of ICM have, at one time or another, consulted headquarters over problems within their country. Sometimes the way forward has been clear. On other occasions considerable time has been spent by both headquarters and the member association in the preparation of background papers, formulation of project proposals, and presentation of a case, usually to the government in respect of legislation or education. Membership associations of ICM are today spread across the world. A majority are within Europe, but the numbers in the African, American, and Asia–Pacific regions are not far behind.

STRUCTURE AND OPERATION OF THE INTERNATIONAL CONFEDERATION OF MIDWIVES

The small, business-like headquarters in London houses the first full-time Secretary-General and her staff. Three times a year the Director (Australia), Deputy Director (United States), and Treasurer (United Kingdom) meet as the Board of Management, responsible for seeing that the policies established at the preceding triennial council meeting are being implemented. An independent expert finance sub-committee offers advice on money management, and progress on the triennial action plan is reviewed in the light of reports from the regions.

In mid-triennium the Executive Committee meets, usually hosted by one of the member associations, to prepare advice for council on the professional policy and philosophy which guides ICM's action. At the Executive Committee meeting held in Madrid, in 1991, the finalized draft of the first *International Code of Ethics* was prepared. The Council voted unanimously to adopt this in May 1993, so giving all midwives a formal, public declaration of their commonly held professional beliefs and values (ICM, 1993).

Council, composed of two representatives from each member association, the 11 Regional Representatives, Officers, and the Board of Management, generally only meets once in each triennium, for 3 days in the week preceding Congress. It is during this meeting that a review of the previous triennium is undertaken, policies revised and agreed, and decisions made for the forthcoming triennium. Board of Management members are elected following nomination by and with the support of their member associations. Other elections select Regional Representatives, two within Africa, two within the Americas, two within Asia–Pacific, and five who work with member associations in the countries of Europe. The role of Regional Representatives is to liaise between the member associations and headquarters, and to arrange at least one regional activity each triennium. Resolutions put to council by member associations are discussed and put to the vote. Those agreed upon are either published as position and/or policy papers or become part of operational policy.

For reasons of simplicity ICM operates within four regions. This is not a neat division and is therefore not without problems. For example, confusion can arise when a country not strictly within Europe is referred to as a European country. ICM functions in three languages, English, French, and Spanish. Simultaneous translation is carried out at council meetings and the plenary sessions at Congress.

MAKING MIDWIVES' VOICES HEARD – LOUD AND CLEAR

As an NGO, ICM works with two United Nations organizations – primarily WHO and UNICEF. Midwives are designated by their member associations as representatives to United Nations Offices on behalf of ICM. These midwives attend meetings at which topics relevant to the role of the midwife or the health and well-being of women and their babies are discussed. Debates in recent years have included the education of the girl child, female genital mutilation, and the distribution of free and low–cost breast-milk substitutes. The reports submitted after these meetings are considered by ICM's Board of Management and decisions taken on subsequent action.

ICM also receives invitations to international meetings organized by a variety of agencies committed to the reproductive health of women and the well-being of their families. Thanks to the system of regional representation, ICM can be present and active in places as far apart as Delhi, Malta, Botswana, and New York. On these occasions midwives rise to the challenge of addressing issues that are technical and social, as well as clinical, and the result can be greater co-operation between the disciplines in working towards the same goal. Increasingly, collaboration with networks representing consumer groups, such as the World Alliance for Breastfeeding Action (WABA), has been fruitful and effective. It is an important way of putting into practice ICM's philosophy that to empower women is to empower midwives.

TODAY – MIDWIFERY, A GLOBAL PARTNERSHIP

With a world-wide surge in interest in midwifery (governments as far apart as Indonesia and the United States of America are engaged in projects to expand and strengthen the profession), ICM continues to play a vital part in providing a focus for the collection and dissemination of information and expertise. It succeeds in the task using very modest resources (Thompson and Walker, 1993). A considerable international network of midwives extends the headquarter's capacity to respond to the many calls for advice, collaboration, and consultancy which come from all over the world. It ensures a midwifery perspective on subjects as diverse as informatics and district hospitals, systems of classification, and ethics.

The need to examine the provision for women's reproductive health requirements into the next millennium and a concern for the mounting maternal mortality figures have resulted in two recent multi-disciplinary WHO groups: the Expert Committee on Maternal and Child Health, and the Study Group on Nursing and Midwifery Beyond the Year 2000. The ICM has played an active part in both (WHO Study Group, 1994).

A further, important tool for ICM's action is a body of position papers which set out succinctly ICM's beliefs with regard to subjects as varied as the place of birth, midwifery research, harmful birth practices, and AIDS. These papers have been used to campaign on contemporary issues from the point of view of the midwife, much as the pre-war resolution on the midwives' commitment to peace was used. The Vancouver Council (May, 1993), for example, issued a statement on women, children, and midwives in situations of war and civil unrest and on the rights of indigenous women and their families.

THE FUTURE

The most recent Executive Committee meeting of ICM took place in Uganda in 1995. It was a time of stock-taking and planning for the future. With so many countries reviewing legislation, the Regional Representatives were able to consider a global overview of the current status and begin to develop a framework of requirements which can be adapted to each region.

To meet the needs of midwives within the African region, a symposium entitled 'Vision with Action – Midwives and Safe Motherhood' was held. This symposium was attended by midwives from 24 countries, 13 of them within Africa. Each midwife went home with a personally developed action plan to be followed up by ICM over the next 2 years.

The next triennial congress of ICM is scheduled for May 1996 in Oslo, Norway, and will offer midwives a new opportunity to share and explore the many changes that are affecting their practice. There will be a new emphasis on enabling midwives to become active in the political processes which are important in achieving equitable health care for women. Some of the concerns expressed by council members at their meeting in 1993 are unlikely to have been resolved. The rising incidence of girls becoming pregnant during their teenage years and the increasing global incidence of HIV and AIDS are two key issues which require vast resources in terms of providing education and, in the latter case, research to achieve a cure.

CONCLUSION

Midwives and mothers have a symbiotic relationship. They need each other and they learn from each other. The midwives of centuries back would wonder at the complexity of the task which is undertaken in the name of the world's midwives by ICM, but perhaps, reading ICM's position statements, particularly the *Code of Ethics*, they would recognize the same concern which they had for the women and babies in their care. Midwives have very rarely been wealthy, or even particularly influential. Their very existence as a distinct profession has often been under threat. Despite this, they have succeeded in establishing, maintaining, and developing their own network of inter-related professional associations world-wide. They are capable of speaking on important issues with a single voice and of working together for improvements in the reproductive health care of women and of their families, as well as for education and practice improvements for midwives themselves. Their capacity to do this, despite repeated setbacks and frequently severely limited resources, has won them the right to a voice in the international arena wherever maternal and child health are discussed.

Midwives are tenacious, practical women. Three-quarters of a century ago they decided that they needed to break out beyond small, local boundaries to share with each other and to strengthen each other as the profession moved into another, more challenging phase of its existence. Now, 75 years further on, the challenges remain, although the social context has changed dramatically. The world still needs its midwives and ICM continues to work to help them face the challenges together. As their new Code of Ethics states so clearly (ICM, 1993):

> *Midwives work with women, supporting their right to participate actively in decisions about their care, and empowering women to speak for themselves on issues affecting the health of women and their families in their culture/society.*

REFERENCES

Australian College of Midwives Incorporated (1992) *Achievement of Safe Motherhood Goals through Education*. Report of the International Confederation of Midwives Asia–Pacific Region pre-congress workshop, Melbourne, Australia, 23–24 March.

Communications of the International Union of Midwives, 1936, **8**: 61.

Communications of the International Union of Midwives, 1939, **10**: 75.

Donnison, J. (1989) *Midwives and Medical Men; A History of Inter-professional Rivalries and Women's Rights*. Historical Publications, London.

FIGO/ICM (1966) *Maternity Care in the World*, 1st edn. International Confederation of Midwives and International Federation of Gynaecology and Obstetrics, London.

FIGO/ICM (1976) *Maternity Care in the World*, 2nd edn. International Confederation of Midwives and International Federation of Gynaecology and Obstetrics, London.

Fildes, V., Marks, L., and Marland, H. (eds) (1992) *Women and Children First – International Maternal and Infant Welfare, 1870–1945*. Routledge, London.

Gélis, J. (1988) *La Sage-femme ou le Médecin; Une Nouvelle Conception de la Vie*. Fayard, Paris.

ICM (1989) *Planning For Action by Midwives – Mobilising Midwifery Personnel for Safe Motherhood*. International Confederation of Midwives, London.

ICM (1990) *Mortalité Maternelle: Les Sages-femmes se Mobilisent*. International Confederation of Midwives, London.

ICM (1992a) *Progress Report on Country Activities following the International Confederation of Midwives Workshop on Enhancing National Midwifery Services*. International Confederation of Midwives, London.

ICM (1992b) *Report on Country Visits Made to Assess Progress on Plans of Action Formulated at an International Confederation of Midwives Workshop on Enhancing National Midwifery Services, held in Burkina Faso, January 1990*. International Confederation of Midwives, London.

ICM (1993) *International Code of Ethics For Midwives*. International Confederation of Midwives, London.

ICM/WHO/FIGO (1990) *The International Definition of a Midwife*, 1st edn. International Confederation of Midwives, London.

ICM/WHO/FIGO (1992) *The International Definition of a Midwife*, 2nd edn. International Confederation of Midwives, London.

ICM/WHO/UNICEF (1987) *Women's Health and the Midwife – A Global Perspective*. Report of a collaborative pre-congress workshop, The Hague, The Netherlands, August 1987, Ref. WHO/MCM/87.5, World Health Organization, Geneva.

ICM/WHO/UNICEF (1990) *Midwifery Education – Action for Safe Motherhood*. Report of a pre-congress workshop, Kobe, Japan, October 1990, Ref. WHO/MCH/91.3, World Health Organization, Geneva.

ICM/WHO/UNICEF (1994) *Midwifery Practice: Measuring, Developing and Mobilising Quality in Care*. Report of a collaborative pre-congress workshop, Vancouver, Canada, May 1993, World Health Organization, Geneva.

Kwast, B.E. (1991) Maternal mortality: The magnitude and the causes. *Midwifery*, **7**: 4–7.

Litoff, J.B. (1986) *The American Midwife Debate. A Source Book on its Modern Origins*. Greenwood Press, London.

Loudon, I. (1992) *Death In Childbirth – An International Study of Maternal Care and Maternal Mortality 1800–1950*. Clarendon, Oxford.

Maclean, G.D. and Tickner, V.J. (1992) A preliminary evaluation of educational material prepared for the Safe Motherhood Initiative educational project. *Midwifery*, **8**: 143–148.

Mahler, H. (1987) *Call To Action*. Part of an address by Dr Mahler at the launch of the Safe Motherhood Initiative, Nairobi. World Health Organization, Geneva.

Marland, H. (ed.) (1993) *The Art of Midwifery – Early Modern Midwives in Europe.* Routledge, London.

Thompson, A. and Walker, J. (1993) International Confederation Of Midwives – Promoting midwifery world-wide. *British Journal of Midwifery,* 1: 42–47.

WHO Expert Committee (1966) *The Midwife In Maternity Care.* WHO Technical Report Series No. 331, World Health Organization, Geneva.

WHO Study Group (1994) *Nursing beyond the Year 2000.* Technical Report Series 842.

CHAPTER

13

The Midwife's Place: An International Comparison of the Status of Midwives

Raymond DeVries

Studies of midwives most often fall into one of the following two categories:

- Description of the state of midwifery in some part of the world.
- Examination of the outcomes of midwifery care.

Both types of inquiries are important to understand the role midwives play in the care of mothers and babies, but the effectiveness of midwife care or the workings of a midwife programme cannot be fully understood unless we first ask how midwifery fits into the society in which it is found. Why is the work of midwives organized in so many different ways? How (and why) has midwifery evolved? How do different organizational structures and cultural systems influence the midwives' niche in the health care system – the way midwives view their profession, how they do their work, how they are viewed by others?

Consideration of these important initial questions will offer a more complete knowledge not only of midwifery, but also of the operation of health care systems. Because nearly all midwives are women, to study the place of midwives helps us understand the import of gender in the occupational structure of medicine. More generally, the story of midwifery demonstrates that medical systems are not rational and predictable applications of science, but are instead social products subject to the influence of structural arrangements and cultural ideas. The promotion of health will not be achieved without a thorough understanding of the social nature of health care.

In order to understand the foundations of midwifery – the way midwifery fits into society – it is necessary to compare the place of midwives in different societies. Several accounts of midwifery around the world are provided by anthropologists, sociologists, and others. To compare these accounts is to be struck by the great diversity in the status of midwives. While midwives share the common tasks of assisting at birth and caring for the health of women, they do *not* share a common status. In some cultures people genuflect and kiss the hand of a midwife when she passes (Sargent, 1982); in other places midwives are seen as 'polluted' (Jeffery *et al.*, 1989); in yet other cultures midwives are accorded the middling status of 'semi-professional'. These accounts also reveal a wide diversity in recruitment, training, styles of practice, the midwife's place in the community and in the medical system, and the rewards of practice. If we organized midwives along a continuum, with those who use all the tools of modern technology at one end and those who are non-technological in orientation at the other, those on the extreme ends of the continuum would not recognize each other as members of the same occupation.

This diversity extends to the terms used to denote a midwife. The World Health Organization (WHO) would like to distinguish midwives from traditional birth attendants. According to WHO, the term 'midwife' should be reserved for those with professional training and formal education. Some cultures make similar distinctions, using different words for indigenous midwives and for formally educated midwives. In some places distinctions are made *among* indigenous midwives, separating those who assist at birth only occasionally from those who assist regularly (Voorhoeve *et al.*, 1984a, 1984b). To settle this confusion, Cosminsky (1976) offers a generic definition:

> *The term midwife refers to a position which has been socially differentiated as a specialized status by the society. Such a person is regarded as a specialist and a professional in her own eyes and by her community.*

The presence of diversity among midwives is also highlighted by the many accounts of midwives that note the ongoing evolution of this occupation. Titles of books and articles call attention to this aspect of midwifery. Consider *Midwives in Passage: The Modernization of Maternity Care* (Benoit, 1991), 'Midwives in transition' (Rothman, 1990), *Labor Pains: Modern Midwives and Home Birth* (Sullivan and Weitz, 1988). Throughout its history the encounters between midwifery and modern culture have changed midwifery, changes that have not been consistent across cultures.

We can begin to understand these diverse manifestations of midwifery if we focus on common factors that influence the occupation. In their study of contemporary midwives in Great Britain, Australia, and New Zealand, Sullivan and Weitz conclude (1988):

> *The current status of midwives in each country is a product not only of physician status and interests but also of economic development, social stratification, government structure, the timing of regulation, the degree of integration with British medicine, and geographic barriers to health care delivery.*

Browner (1989) provides a comparable list:

> *The social position of midwives varies according to the status of women in society; the status of healers who are not midwives; the amount of technical or other skill that midwives possess, including whether they are responsible for complicated deliveries or whether in such cases they are expected to call upon the other specialists; and whether midwives are chosen by divine selection, self-selection, inheritance, or in other ways.*

These rather long lists of influences on midwifery can be reduced to four factors:

- Geography.
- Technology.
- The structure of society (included here are occupational structures and the arrangements between medical organizations and other institutions – political, legal, economic, religious, educational).
- The culture (meanings and values) of the people served by the midwife.

These categories overlap. Technology is to a certain extent the product of the interaction between culture and structure. And the meanings given to gender (a cultural variable) have a great influence on the way occupations are arranged (a structural variable). Note that technology and geography are physical things that influence the way midwives work. Social structure and culture are less tangible, but no less important, influences on midwifery.

In the following pages, the impacts of technology, social structure, and culture on midwifery are considered. This is not to underestimate the influence of geography. Geographic factors play an important role in the transmission of technology and culture. Many researchers describe the way geographic barriers allow for the survival of pockets of traditional midwifery in modernizing nations. Sullivan and Weitz (1988) detail the ways the geography of New Zealand and Australia influenced the spread of regulation and the practice of midwifery there. Benoit (1991) makes similar observations about granny midwives in rural Canada. In the United States, granny midwives persisted in the rural south largely because of geographic isolation. Geographic factors also figure prominently in Hingstman's (1994) analysis of the survival of a strong profession of midwifery in the Netherlands: he claims that easy access to hospitals found in this small, flat country makes safe the continued use of midwife-assisted home birth. But further analysis of this phenomenon is beyond the scope of this paper and is best left to medical geographers.

TECHNOLOGY

For better or worse, technology changes the character and the meaning of work. Essayist Wendell Berry (1990) calls our attention to this fact when he explains his refusal to use a personal computer. He is certain that the move from pencil and typewriter to computer will diminish his relationships with his editor, his typist, and the local community. Unlike most of us, he is unwilling to make that sacrifice.

The history of midwifery suggests that Berry is right. Technology has changed, and continues to change, midwifery. It is conventional wisdom that midwifery forceps were the 'technological breakthrough' that led to the decline of midwifery in most Western nations. But how does technology diminish midwifery? It is obvious that midwives suffer because they lack access to new tools and techniques, but this is just part of the story. New (and successful) technology challenges the legitimacy and authority of midwifery. As technology replaces tradition, patterns of recruitment are changed and doubts about existing techniques, definitions, and sources of knowledge that surround birth are created.

In traditional societies a midwife's authority comes from her 'call' (see, for example, Cosminsky, 1976; Buss, 1980; MacCormack, 1982; Laderman 1983). Traditional midwives become midwives because of a 'call' that is either supernatural or through tradition (i.e., biological or social heredity). Their training follows from this 'call', from the hands of another experienced and accepted midwife or, occasionally, in the form of visions or dreams. Technology changes this traditional pattern. In technological societies recruitment is not the basis of legitimacy. No one is concerned with the reasons a midwife chooses her occupation. Training and certification are the primary sources of authority. As Cosminsky (1982) notes, "training is offered as an alternative to a divine mandate, opening up the role to others who want to practise."

Technology brings in its wake ideas, definitions, and approaches to childbirth that supplant traditional patterns. Laderman (1983) calls our attention to the way technology alters concepts of 'trained' and 'untrained':

> Every active village midwife [in rural Malaysia] ... has been fully trained ....
> Characterizing bidan kampung [local midwives] as untrained is an expression of
> cultural bias in favor of formal schooling over apprenticeship. It is not an
> objective description of fact.

WHO shares this technological bias when it observes that "two-thirds of the babies in the world are delivered without a *trained* attendant." This statement invalidates all non-formal modes of education (Cosminsky 1976).

Formal training discounts *all* other sources of knowledge, including traditional midwifery and the unique information a client possesses (about her body, previous births, etc.). This attitude is evident to traditional midwives in Benin. Sargent (1989) reports that a midwife there:

> would have appreciated learning from clinic staff and had hoped to work together,
> as in the past, when the indigenous midwife would accompany her client to the
> dispensary in the event of complications. Now, she said, the 'heart' of the nurses is
> unwelcoming.

In their collection of statistics on childbirth in rural Kenya, Voorhoeve *et al.* (1984a) demonstrate this lack of faith in the knowledge of indigenous midwives. Note the tone of the following comment (emphasis added): "none of the midwives ever *admitted* that any of their patients had a total perineal tear." Specialized instruments and machinery "provide a kind of knowledge of the event that is privileged" (Jordan and Irwin, 1987).

Kirkham (1986) summarizes the tremendous impact of technology on midwifery:

> Previously all pregnancies were seen as normal until judged otherwise, a
> judgement usually made initially by a midwife. The reverse is now true, as all
> pregnancies now fall under medical management and are 'normal only in
> retrospect'. By this logic the midwife as practitioner in her own right is defined out
> of existence.

The possibility of being 'defined out of existence' is very real. Unlike other traditional healers, who can find a niche in modern medical systems by treating native diseases peculiar to their area (diseases outside the ken of modern medicine), indigenous midwives find their services exactly duplicated by other 'modern' birth attendants. For this reason Laderman (1983) is concerned about the future of traditional midwives in Malaysia. Technology is able to create a uniform culture and this is a culture that makes midwifery obsolete. Jordan (1987; see also Jordan, 1989) makes the interesting observation that the instruments of high technology are more portable between cultures than are indigenous, low technology items:

> *Although one imports a fetal monitor to do electronic fetal monitoring, it would not make sense to import ropes from Africa so that women could hold onto them during labor.*

Technological culture seems able to overwhelm other cultural influences. Holland and McKevitt (1985) suspected that childbirth in the former Soviet Union might be more humane and tender because the majority of Soviet physicians are female. They hypothesized that the nurturing values learned by little girls might translate into more gentle care than that given by the male dominated profession of obstetrics in Western nations. But they discovered this was not the case. The former Soviet Union had a technologically advanced system in which the few remaining midwives serve as obstetric nurses. Labouring women were treated much as they would be in any hospital: often left alone and forced to fit their labours into the hospital schedule. The hegemony of technology, the unwillingness to consider other sources of knowledge, is evident in this statement by a Soviet physician (Holland and McKevitt, 1985, emphasis added):

> *The doctor cannot put the question of the desirability of this or that therapeutic measure before the woman in labour and establish this right to choose treatment measures. You see, if we establish this right for women in labour then, whether we like it or not, it automatically shifts responsibility for the outcome of the birth onto the child-bearing woman.* **Therefore such a position is incorrect**.

When technology is applied to birth, the experience is redefined in terms of differing levels of risk. Sophisticated instruments of detection allow every birth to be defined in terms of the risk for an undesired outcome. The attraction of technology is thereby increased because it promises to reduce the risks of birth. Once the language of risk is established, it allows physicians to decide which births can be safely handled by midwives. Kaufert and O'Neil (1993) noticed this among an Inuit settlement in Canada:

> *The epidemiological language of risk determines the medical view, and this medical view – as expressed by the physician – determines obstetric policy ... the medical profession relies on arguments of risk to the fetus to elicit compliance by individual women [and] to persuade the government to invest in obstetric care.*

The increasing tendency to define all births in terms of 'risk' (low or high) has a profound impact on the profession of midwifery, allowing the definer(s) of risk to determine the workload of midwives and creating an image of midwives in the minds of the public. This relationship between risk and midwifery is explored more fully later, in the conclusion.

SOCIAL STRUCTURE

Although it is somewhat artificial to separate culture and structure, it is useful to look at the ways that social structure influences midwives. Most important for our analysis is the organization of the system that delivers health care and its relation to other parts of the society. In some societies midwives are a regular and accepted part of the health care delivery system. In other places midwives either do not exist or play only a marginal role.

In her comparison of the roles of midwives in five Western countries (Sweden, the Netherlands, Britain, United States, Canada), Benoit (forthcoming) distinguishes 'midwifery' and 'medical' models of care. According to Benoit, the health care systems of Sweden and the Netherlands have midwifery models of care that allow midwives to play an important and independent role (see also Van Teijlingen, 1990; Abraham-van der mark, 1993; Hingstman, forthcoming). Britain, the United States, and Canada have medical models of childbirth care. In the medical model midwives have little autonomy and often function as assistants.

Why do these differences exist? The success of midwifery as an autonomous occupation is closely tied to the structural arrangements for the payment of services. Decisions by governments and private insurance companies determine the terms of existence for midwives. It is informative to contrast the situations of midwives in three countries that have national health insurance: Britain, Sweden, and the Netherlands. Sullivan and Weitz (1988) comment on the effect of the establishment of the National Health Service (NHS) in England in 1946:

> The immediate effect of the NHS was to discourage the dwindling number of independent, fee-for-service, midwives in Britain. These women could not compete with the free care provided by the government. The NHS not only removed the cost differential between midwives and physicians, but also removed the economic barrier that kept many high-risk, low-income mothers out of hospitals. In addition, the program paid general practitioners for obstetric cases whether or not they attended the delivery. The latter provision created a resurgence of interest in routine prenatal care among general practitioners.

In Sweden, because of the creation of a decentralized maternity care system, midwifery is not diminished by nationalized health care. Most maternity care is provided at 'mothercare centres' staffed by midwives. Complicated cases are referred by midwives to general practitioners at 'Type II Clinics' or to obstetricians at 'Type-III Clinics'. The Dutch also have a decentralized maternity system that promotes independent midwifery. In the Netherlands, midwives are remunerated on a fee-for-service system and are allowed to supervise normal deliveries at home and in hospitals.

The author's study (DeVries, 1996) of midwives in the United States and the Netherlands underscores the importance of insurance plans for midwives. Government recognition in the form of a license does not guarantee the flourishing of midwifery. A midwife might be licensed, but if insurance companies do not pay for her services her viability is uncertain. In a few American states 'lay' midwives (i.e., non-nurse midwives) are allowed to practise, but where they are unable to be reimbursed by insurance companies, they remain marginal. By contrast, the *Ziekenfondswet* (Sick Funds law), established in 1941 in the Netherlands, gives the

Dutch midwife a *primaat*: if midwife care is available and if a women is expected to have a 'normal' birth, the state system of health insurance will not pay for care by a physician. This advantage in the market place has allowed midwives in the Netherlands to remain an important part of maternity care. Parenthetically, this relationship between insurance and midwives in the United States could work in favour of the occupation. With the coming 'corporatization of medical care' (Starr, 1982; McKinley and Stoeckle, 1988), insurance companies, looking for more economic approaches to health care, might begin to favour the services of midwives (DeClercq, 1992).

The structure of the midwives' work-setting also influences the nature of her practice. Benoit (forthcoming) suggests that, even though midwives in Sweden and the Netherlands have a great deal of independence, their different work settings create very different types of midwifery. In particular, she claims that the professional status of Dutch midwives is hindered by the fee-for-service system because it isolates midwives, requires them to compete for clients, provides little opportunity for career advancement, and forces them into an unpredictable round-the-clock work schedule. By way of contrast, Sweden's midwives have regular hours, a steady flow of clients, interaction with colleagues, and well-defined career ladders. Benoit (1989b) also provides an analysis of the way levels of bureaucratization are related to midwife practice. She concludes that a middle level of bureaucracy, as represented by cottage hospitals in Newfoundland and Labrador (Canada), provides the most freedom for midwives' practices.

Political structure plays a part in the fate of midwifery. Government regulations that control the practices of midwives are hammered out in political settings. Several researchers have commented on the easy legislative access American physicians have by virtue of their professional associations and the significant sums of money spent on lobbying and campaign contributions. In her analysis of the failed attempt of Colorado's lay midwives to secure the right to practise in that state, Tjaden (1987) notes:

> Lay midwives have neither a professional lobbyist nor a national affiliation that can be used to apply political pressure in the Colorado legislature ...[lay midwives do] not contribute money to political campaigns, nor can [they] promise very many votes to legislators.

In the author's research of midwifery in four states, a close relationship was observed between the professional organizations of physicians and the governmental bodies charged with regulating health care professions (DeVries, 1985). Such influence is more difficult in other political systems. In the Netherlands – where midwives still maintain independent practices – the structure of the electoral system and the Dutch tradition of a great number of representative advisory councils make it more difficult for physicians (or any group) to influence legislation.

The place of midwifery is dependent on educational structures. The degree of independence midwives have is directly related to the nature of their education: its content and the qualifications of those who do the teaching. When midwives learn from other midwives, in apprenticeship systems or in vocational schools, a separate body of 'midwife knowledge' is kept alive and so midwives are equipped to work independently. When midwives are instructed by members of other occupational groups (physicians or nurses), they are more likely to work as assistants to other professions. Benoit (1989a) looked at the relation between educational background and practices of midwives in rural areas of Canada. She noted that midwives who are academically trained, under the "continuous supervision of medical specialists and hospital bureaucrats," have a 'narrow occupational role'; while midwives trained in vocational schools score higher on 'professional status', and are able to operate with "a substantial degree of freedom from community and bureaucratic control."

The larger social structure also affects midwifery. For instance, opportunities afforded by the occupational structure can influence the flow of women into midwifery. Sargent (1989) observed this in Benin, where becoming a midwife was a route to enhanced prestige for women. But with modernization, many other avenues for prestige enhancement became open to young women. She goes on to point out that this fact and other structural and cultural forces (government policies, the need for certified birth certificates unavailable from traditional midwives, and increasing scorn and harassment of home-birth women) are directing women away from using and becoming indigenous midwives:

> Although maternity remains central to the concept of the successful woman, the accretion of other possibilities in the public domain, such as salaried worker, provide alternatives – both symbolic and actual – to traditionally acceptable options, principally that of midwife.

CULTURE

How does culture influence the acceptance of midwifery as a practice and as a system of belief about women and birth? It is no exaggeration to say that midwifery will not long survive if it does not 'make sense' in terms of the local culture. A midwife's place in society is affected by cultural ideas about pregnancy and birth, about the role of women, about religion, and about technology.

Perhaps the clearest example of culture's influence on midwives is found in India. The religious system there specifies that the touching of bodily fluids is 'polluting'. Given the fact that a birth attendant inevitably comes into contact with bodily fluids, the status of an Indian midwife (known as a *dāi*) is very low. In fact, Jeffery *et al.* (1989) suggest *dāis* should not be known as midwives:

> It is inappropriate to regard the dāi as an expert midwife in the contemporary Western sense. Even in the absence of medically trained personnel, the dāi does not have overriding control over the management of deliveries. Nor is she a sisterly and supportive equal. Rather, she is a low status menial necessary for removing defilement.

The author's study (DeVries, 1985) of lay midwives in several states in the United States also revealed connections between religion and midwifery. Religious beliefs were often a primary factor in seeking the services of a midwife. For example, many Jehovah's Witnesses, anxious to avoid hospital procedures that violated their beliefs (e.g., they believe that it is wrong to accept a blood transfusion), solicited the services of lay midwives for home births. Religious groups, when correctly situated, can influence legislation. A legislator in Arizona, one of few states where lay midwives gained the legal right to practise, explained that a large Mormon constituency with a preference for midwife-attended home birth 'encouraged' a positive vote on the part of many members of the legislature.

Secular values can have a similar effect on legislation. In explaining the success of a bill that favoured lay midwives in New Hampshire, a midwife pointed to the Yankee tradition of independence and self-reliance. In the state whose automobile license plates proclaim, 'Live Free or Die', it would seem incongruous to deny the freedom for midwife-attended home birth. She claimed that a group of wizened old Yankee men (most born at home themselves) were not about to let the representatives of medical organizations deny this basic freedom to New Hampshire citizens.

Cultural values determine the nature of the midwife's role and the prestige it possesses. Browner (1989) says that few women in the village of San Francisco in Oaxaca choose to become midwives. Why? Because "the role offers little advantage." Information on childbirth is widely shared, families attend their own births, and consequently midwives have little 'esoteric' knowledge.

Ideas about gender and the role of women in the occupational structure – important for midwives and all women working outside the home – are rooted in culture. Because midwifery is an occupation dominated by women, it is more easily subject to incursions from other professional groups. Radosh (1986) finds this a crucial factor in the demise of American midwifery in the early twentieth century:

> The sex roles of the period relegated women to non-professional spheres by definition ... the fact that the profession was female-dominated, and thus low status, assured that usual professional concerns for economic, social or political viability were not salient ...

Culture also plays an important part in the relation between midwives and clients. Sargent (1982) notes:

> Clients and indigenous midwives [in Benin] are found to be homophilous in that they share concepts of causation, beliefs, values and role expectations.

She goes on to point out that the absence of homophily deters prospective clients from using the obstetric services of government-provided nurse-midwives. These practitioners do not share the world view of their clients, often speak to them only in French, and are quick to criticize client behaviour.

The situation is the same in many other locations. In Ghana, Eades *et al.* (1993) observed women seeking traditional birth attendants because they share "similar beliefs, values, and ideas about the cause of illness," and avoiding hospitals because of the "expectation of disrespectful or painful treatment." Kamal (1992) notes that in India, the "traditional birth attendant [*dāi*] enjoys greater confidence within the community than the modern registered midwife; her ways are not alien to the family." In her study of midwives in Malaysia, Laderman (1983) describes a similar process. In one village, a government-provided midwife, unfamiliar with the local culture, had an uneasy relationship with the residents she served. But (and this is an important *but*), Laderman noticed this midwife was respected for her knowledge of, and connections to, the bureaucracy. She was especially valued because she was the only one who could summon the ambulance in emergencies. Laderman's study reminds us of the subtle ways culture can change. Local culture was powerful enough to make an 'outside midwife' feel out of place, but not powerful enough to resist the new definitions and new possibilities offered by this midwife. The villagers distrusted the government midwife, but they recognized the utility of her view of birth and her treatments and valued access to 'her' technology. Gradually, the 'taken for granted' definitions of birth change.

Cultural change can promote midwifery. The renaissance of independent midwifery in the United States (and to a lesser extent in Canada) in the 1960s and 1970s offers an example of cultural change encouraging a revival of traditional birth techniques. The nearly simultaneous emergence of the anti-Vietnam war movement, the civil rights movement, the feminist movement, and the ecology movement called into question a number of American cultural values and challenged all forms of institutionalized authority. Rothman (1990) asserts that the 'rights orientation' that emerged in the mid-1960s "dramatically reduced the discretionary authority of a number of social actors." This was certainly true in medicine, where many questioned the institutionalization and 'medicalization' of birth. As a result of this cultural change, independent midwives flourished in several areas and there was a small but significant rise in home births (DeVries, 1984; Reid, 1989; Rushing, 1993).

STRUCTURE AND CULTURE

Structure and culture interact in significant ways to shape the practice of midwifery. For example, consider the fate of midwifery in the United States, where the disintegration of midwifery was quite rapid. Physicians were able to exploit their structural advantage (i.e., connections to the political system) to promote legislation that eliminated or effectively reduced the practice of midwifery (Devitt, 1979; DeVries, 1985). This structural advantage created a cultural advantage. Denied the credibility of licenses, midwives lost their place in the reimbursement system and gradually lost their legitimacy in the eyes of the public. The structural advantage that allowed physicians to promote legislation that prohibited midwifery also allowed them to modify the cultural definition of midwives. Where once midwives were the only birth attendant women trusted, now they are defined as ill-trained, dirty, and dangerous. Hospital birth, once considered odd, is now 'safer', 'more fashionable', 'easier'. The structural and cultural advantage of physician organizations remains visible in those states where lay midwives are seeking licensure. Susie (1988) describes the situation in the state of Florida, where physicians used their political and economic influence to overturn a 1982 law that allowed licenses to lay midwives.

Laderman's (1983) study of Malaysian midwives offers a good example of the interaction between the occupational structure of a society and its culture. She observes that in some areas the availability of a government midwife reduced the duties of the traditional midwife to:

> *Laundry, cooking, cleaning, bathing the baby, and massaging the mother.*
> *Stripped of her obstetric role and reduced to the status of household help, the traditional bidan's calling will no longer ring so loudly in the ears of the village girls.*

As technology influences the work of the midwife, the meaning of the occupation changes and it becomes a less attractive one.

The interaction of culture and structure can also be seen in the rise of alternative birth settings in the United States. The cultural challenge presented to the medicalization of birth in the 1960s and 1970s resulted in structural changes in the delivery of care in childbirth. The new meanings given birth (as 'natural', not 'medical'; as a family experience, an opportunity for 'bonding') caused associations of medical professionals to recommend change and to endorse nurse-midwives. Hospitals responded by creating new environments for birth and by hiring nurse-midwives to staff them. Providers of health care equipment contributed to this change by mounting marketing campaigns to sell products designed for these new birth environments. The Borning Corporation has a well crafted presentation on 'natural birth' intended to promote sales of a bed made to facilitate combined labour and delivery rooms in hospitals.

MIDWIFERY AS A PROFESSION: RISK, KNOWLEDGE, AND POWER

Our analysis of midwifery leaves us with a final question: Can midwives survive in the modern world – with its technology, university models of education, complicated health insurance schemes – without sacrificing their tradition, their identity, and their unique body of knowledge? To answer this question we must consider two things:

- The structural, cultural, and technological constraints that operate on midwives.
- The way midwives wish to define their profession in a changing medical culture.

How does the 'culture of midwifery' suit it for survival in the midst of cultural and social change? The essence of midwifery is low-technology, one-to-one supportive care. When midwives reflect on their tradition, they celebrate the simple and practical wisdom of their forebears. But this low-technology tradition is not ideally suited to the modern world. By way of contrast, consider the more pragmatic culture of allopathic medicine. When allopaths look back on their forebears, whose therapies (e.g., bleeding and purging) would now be seen as 'quackery', they celebrate the *pragmatic spirit* embodied there. The culture of midwifery stresses being *practical* and *simple*, the culture of medicine stresses being *pragmatic*.

Being practical and simple does not necessarily help an occupational group survive societal change. For example, the wisdom of midwifery suggests that only one who is 'called' should become a midwife; several lay midwife groups in the United States, when establishing criteria for programmes for midwifery credentials, made some effort to ascertain the reasons for pursuing this occupation. This makes practical sense. Those who are called have a reason to withstand the hardships of midwifery; they have a larger sense of the importance of their task. Buss (1980) illustrates the way a call translates into commitment when she describes the tireless Jesusita, a *partera* in rural New Mexico, who attended the births of 11,924 babies and is willing to care for women who cannot pay her. But this approach to recruitment is not pragmatic. It does not ensure 'enough' midwives, it does not promote the profession, it does not ensure that all candidates have certain 'standard' qualifications, and, in societies that equate technological mastery with credibility, it does not establish midwifery as a credible occupation.

In thinking about the survival of midwifery (or any profession) it is important to recognize that at least three different types of interests are at stake:

- The interests of midwives as *persons.*
- The interests of midwifery as a *profession.*
- The interests of midwifery as a *service* (interested in the health and well-being of women and babies).

It is too often assumed that all three of these are of one piece, that an improvement in any one brings an improvement in all the others. This has been the assumption of physicians: "What is good for us (personally and professionally) is good for our clients." But this is decidedly not true. Often, the interests of the profession are at odds with the interests of clients and often the maintenance of a strong profession puts heavy demands on members of the profession.

In the Netherlands the organization of midwifery care has been good for the profession of midwifery. Advocates of midwifery in the United States point to the Netherlands as a model for midwifery care. They note that Dutch midwives have a good deal of autonomy, that they are free to work with little supervision. But these situations are not good for midwives as persons. The hours are gruelling and family life becomes impossible (Jabaaij, 1994). In Sweden, midwives as persons benefit from the government organization of midwifery clinics – hours are regular and predictable and they have a certain degree of autonomy. But the independent profession of midwifery is compromised; they are not as free as their colleagues in the Netherlands.

And what of the third element: the interests of clients? Where are clients best served? If the criterion of choice is used, clients are best served by a more autonomous profession because it offers a choice between *true* alternatives. In places like the Netherlands, clients have the opportunity to benefit from the independent tradition of midwifery. In places where midwives have gained legitimacy by affiliation with technological medicine, clients have less choice. Midwife care looks much like physician care. In the long run clients benefit from having more than one medical tradition. When strong and vital approaches to health care can interact, they learn from each other. There are several instances in which physicians learned valuable techniques from midwives, including approaches to avoiding perineal tears and the importance of immediate contact between parents and babies (DeVries, 1984).

Many midwives believe that it is in the best interests of midwifery to define itself as a 'profession'. What makes an occupation a profession? Must midwifery establish itself as a profession to survive? Reid (1989) suggests that midwifery is best thought of as a 'semi-profession', because it has some of the trademarks of a profession, but lacks all the features:

> *Although [midwives] work with some independence, they are restricted from attending high-risk labors and deliveries and from using a number of medical technologies. Ultimately they are accountable to others, most notably, physicians.*

Social scientists disagree about the defining features of a profession. Some claim a list of traits (prolonged training, a professional association, a code of ethics, etc.)

separates a profession from other occupations. Others assert that there is one defining feature of a profession: power (Abbott, 1988, for a summary of this literature). Our analysis of the varied statuses of midwives helps us rethink the criteria that establish an occupational group as a profession.

I suggest that an occupational group gains power to the extent that it can reduce risk and uncertainty for clients. Doctors are valued because they help their clients deal with sickness, an unscheduled and uncertain status transition. Lawyers gain prestige and power because they handle unnerving and uncertain problems, such as divorce and litigations that threaten our material well-being. Members of the clergy help people deal with the uncertain fate of their souls. The most highly rewarded members of society (in terms of money, prestige, and power) are those that reduce the most frightening risks. In a less secular age, priests were the most important risk reducers and were among the most powerful members of society. Today our concerns are more existential, our bodies and our material possessions are more important than our souls; hence physicians and lawyers are the primary risk reducers.

My thesis suggests that professional groups can gain power by 'creating' risk – that is by *emphasizing* risk, highlighting uncertainty, by redefining life events as 'risky'. Perhaps the best example of this is the promotion of prenuptial contracts by lawyers, intended to avoid the risks of divorce. Medicine encourages us to see once-normal life experiences, including eating, exercise, and ageing, as fraught with risk.

We can understand the occupational status of midwives by considering the way they relate to risk. How do midwives gain power (status, prestige, and respect)? Cross-cultural study shows that midwives are respected to the extent that they can offer some way (be it technological, spiritual, or some combination of these) to reduce risk and uncertainty. Although birth has a more regular and predictable trajectory than sickness, it is nevertheless a risky event, especially in traditional societies where mortality rates are high. Where they are the primary managers of the risk of birth, midwives have high status. Where other practitioners offer 'better' means of risk reduction *or* where births are categorized according to their level of risk and midwives are only allowed to assist at those defined by others as 'low' risk, midwives lose status. Landy (1978) notes that the traditional healer's role faces the greatest challenge:

> as the course of disease becomes more controllable (prevention, public health
> measures), more predictable (medical intervention with miracle drugs, scientific
> surgery), and less uncertain.

Midwives were bound to lose status as they were limited to assisting at 'low-risk births' and as other, 'better', practitioners appeared who could help manage this uncertain time. By the same logic, obstetricians enhance their status by increasing the number of surgical deliveries (i.e., caesarean sections) that they perform.

Gender is a factor here. In most societies, women care for the sick. But the care they give is palliative care. They are a presence during the uncertain episodes of sickness, but they do not alter its course or reduce its impact through intervention. Historically, men often played the more 'heroic' role (with all its good and bad connotations) with regard to sickness. Their ministrations were seen as reducers of uncertainty, as the hope of salvation. This is how midwifery forceps were perceived when they were introduced by the Chamberlens in the seventeenth century. Midwives, whose less interventionist tradition led them to eschew forceps, became less desirable attendants.

This analysis of the relationship between risk and professional status leads to the unfortunate conclusion that the attempt by some midwives to seek a niche in modern medical systems by claiming to be experts in 'low-risk' birth threatens their credibility as a professional group. Prestige and power are given to those who manage high-risk situations, not to those who attend to low-risk births. But midwives face an unusual predicament: to enhance their status it seems they must renounce their tradition. They can earn their niche in the system only if they cease to be recognizable as midwives.

In seeking to survive, midwives must ask: survive for whom? For the good of the profession? For their own good as practitioners? Or for the health of the women and babies they serve?

ACKNOWLEDGEMENT

This chapter is a revised version of an article first published in Riska and Wegar (1993), used by permission of the author and Sage Publications. This research was supported in part by a grant (FO6-TW01954) from the Fogarty Center of the National Institutes of Health (US) and by NIVEL (Netherlands Institute for the Study of Primary Health Care).

REFERENCES

Abbott, A. (1988) *The System of the Professions.* University of Chicago Press, Chicago.

Abraham-van der mark, E. (ed.) (1993) *Successful Home Birth and Midwifery: The Dutch Model.* Bergin and Garvey, London.

Benoit, C. (1989a) The professional socialisation of midwives: Balancing art and science. *Sociology of Health and Illness,* **11**(2): 160–180.

Benoit, C. (1989b) Traditional midwifery practice: The limits of occupational autonomy. *Canadian Review of Sociology and Anthropology,* **26**(4): 633–649.

Benoit, C. (1991) *Midwives in Passage: The Modernization of Maternity Care.* ISER Books, St. John's, Newfoundland.

Berry, W. (1990) *What are People For?* North Point Press, San Francisco.

Browner, C.H. (1989) The management of reproduction in an egalitarian society. In: McClain, C.S. (ed.), *Women as Healers: Cross-Cultural Perspectives.* Rutgers, New Brunswick, NJ.

Buss, F.L. (1980) *La Partera, Story of a Midwife.* The University of Michigan Press, Ann Arbor.

Cosminsky, S. (1976) Cross-cultural perspectives on midwifery. In: Grollig, F.X. and Haley, H.B. (eds), *Medical Anthropology.* Mouton, The Hague.

Cosminsky, S. (1982) Childbirth and change: A Guatemalan study. In: MacCormack, C.P. (ed.), *Ethnography of Fertility and Birth.* Academic Press, New York.

DeClercq, E. (1992) The transformation of American midwifery: 1975 to 1988. *American Journal of Public Health,* **82**: 680–684.

Devitt, N. (1979) How doctors conspired to eliminate the midwife even though scientific data supported midwifery. In: Stewart, D. and Stewart, L. (eds), *Compulsory Hospitalization or Freedom of Choice in Childbirth?* NAPSAC, Marble Hill, MO.

DeVries, R. (1984) Humanizing childbirth: The discovery and implementation of bonding theory. *International Journal of Health Services,* **14**(1): 89–104.

DeVries, R. (1985) *Regulating Birth: Midwives, Medicine and the Law.* Temple University Press, Philadelphia.

DeVries, R. (1996) Midwives among the machines: Recreating midwifery in the twentieth century. In: Rafferty, A.M. and Marland, H. (eds), *Midwives and Society: 1850 to the Present.* Routledge, London.

Eades, C., Brace, C., Osei, L., and LaGuardia, K. (1993) Traditional birth attendants and maternal mortality in Ghana. *Social Science and Medicine,* **36**(11): 1503–1507.

Hingstman, L. (1994) Primary care obstetrics and perinatal health in the Netherlands. *Journal of Nurse-Midwifery* , **39**: 379–386.

Holland, B. and McKevitt, T. (1985) Maternity care in the Soviet Union. In: Holland, B. (ed.), *Soviet Sisterhood.* Indiana University Press, Bloomington.

Jabaaij, L. (1994) *De Vrijgevestigde Verloskundige in Nederland; Werk and Werkdruk (The Independent Midwife in the Netherlands: Work and Workload).* NIVEL, Utrecht, the Netherlands.

Jeffery, P., Jeffery, R., and Lyon, A. (1989) *Labour Pains and Labour Power: Women and Childbearing in India.* Zed Books, London.

Jordan, B. (1987) The hut and the hospital: Information, power and symbolism in the artifacts of birth. *Birth,* **14**(1): 36–40.

Jordan, B. (1989) Cosmopolitical obstetrics: Some insights from the training of traditional midwives. *Social Science and Medicine,* **28**(9): 925–944.

Jordan, B. and Irwin, S. (1987) A close encounter with a court-ordered cesarean section: A case of differing realities. In: Baer, H.A. (ed.), *Encounters with Biomedicine.* Gordon & Breach, New York.

Kamal, I.T. (1992) The traditional birth attendant. *World Health,* Sept–Oct: 6–7.

Kaufert, P. and O'Neil, J. (1993) Analysis of a dialogue on the risks of childbirth. In: Lindebaum, S. and Lock, M. (eds), *Knowledge, Power, and Practice: The Anthropology of Medicine and Everyday Life.* University of California Press, Berkeley.

Kirkham, M. (1986) A feminist perspective in midwifery. In: Webb, C. (ed.), *Feminist Practice in Women's Health Care.* John Wiley & Sons, New York.

Laderman, C. (1983) *Wives and Midwives: Childbirth and Nutrition in Rural Malaysia.* University of California, Berkeley.

Landy, D. (1978) Role adaptation: traditional curers under the impact of Western medicine. In: Logan, M.H. and Hunt, E.E. (eds.), *Health and the Human Condition.* Duxbury, North Scituate, MA.

MacCormack, C.P. (1982) Biological, cultural and social adaptation in human fertility and birth: A synthesis. In: MacCormack, C.P. (ed.), *Ethnography of Fertility and Birth.* Academic Press, New York.

McKinley, J. and Stoeckle, J. (1988) Corporation and the social transformation of doctoring. *International Journal of Health Services,* **18**(2): 191–205.

Radosh, P.F. (1986) Midwives in the United States: Past and present. *Population Research and Policy Review,* **5**: 129–145.

Reid, M. (1989) Sisterhood and professionalization: A case study of the American lay midwife. In: McClain, C.S. (ed.), *Women as Healers: Cross-Cultural Perspectives.* Rutgers, New Brunswick, NJ.

Riska, E. and Wegar, E. (eds) (1993) *Gender, Work and Medicine.* Sage, London.

Rothman, B.K. (1983) Midwives in transition: The structure of a clinical revolution. *Social Problems,* **30**(3): 262–271.

Rothman, D. (1990) Human experimentation and the origins of bioethics. In: Weisz, G. (ed.), *Social Science Perspectives on Medical Ethics.* Kluwer Academic Publishers, Dordrecht.

Rushing, B. (1993) Ideology and the reemergence of North American midwifery. *Work and Occupations,* **20**(1): 46–67.

Sargent, C. (1982) *The Cultural Context of Therapeutic Choice: Obstetrical Care Decisions among the Bariba of Benin.* D. Reidel, Dordrecht.

Sargent, C. (1989) Women's roles and women healers in contemporary rural and urban Benin. In: McClain, C.S. (ed.), *Women as Healers: Cross-Cultural Perspectives.* Rutgers, New Brunswick, NJ.

Starr, P. (1982) *The Social Transformation of American Medicine.* Basic Books, New York.

Sullivan, D. and Weitz, R. (1988) *Labor Pains: Modern Midwives and Home Birth.* Yale, New Haven.

Susie, D.A. (1988) *In the Way of Our Grandmothers: A Cultural View of Twentieth-Century Midwifery in Florida.* University of Georgia Press, Athens, GA.

Tjaden, P.G. (1987) Midwifery in Colorado: A case study in the politics of professionalization. *Qualitative Sociology,* **10**(1): 29–45.

Van Teijlingen, E. (1990) The profession of maternity home care assistant and its significance for the Dutch midwifery profession. *International Journal of Nursing Studies,* **27**(4): 355–366.

Voorhoeve, A.M., Kars, C., and van Ginneken, J.K. (1984a) Modern and traditional antenatal and delivery care. In: van Ginneken, J.K. and Muller, A.S. (eds), *Maternal and Child Health in Rural Kenya.* Croom Helm, London.

Voorhoeve, A.M., Kars, C., and van Ginneken, J.K. (1984b) The outcome of pregnancy. In: van Ginneken, J.K. and Muller, A.S. (eds), *Maternal and Child Health in Rural Kenya.* Croom Helm, London.

Index